NURSING ASSIGNMENT PATTERNS
USER'S MANUAL

NURSING ASSIGNMENT PATTERNS USER'S MANUAL

Fred C. Munson
Joanne Shultz Beckman
Jacqueline Clinton
Carolyn Kever
Lillian M. Simms

AUPHA PRESS
Ann Arbor, Michigan • Washington, D.C.
1980

Library of Congress Cataloging in Publication Data

Main entry under title:

Nursing assignment patterns.

Includes bibliographies.
1. Nursing service administration—Problems, exercises, etc. I. Munson, Fred C. [DNLM: 1. Nursing staff, Hospital—Organ. 2. Nursing service, Hospital—Organ. WY105 N9743]
RT 89.N79   610.73'068'3   80-12014

ISBN 0-914904-40-X pbk.

80 81 82 83 84/6 5 4 3 2 1

AUPHA Press is an imprint within Health Administration Press.

Health Administration Press
School of Public Health
University of Michigan
Ann Arbor, Michigan 48109

313-764-1380

AUPHA Press
One DuPont Circle
Washington, D.C. 20036

202-659-4354

ACKNOWLEDGMENTS

This manual represents the results of efforts of many people. The original idea evolved from discussions between Barbara Horn, Barbara Lee and Fred Munson about elements of a framework developed by Barbara Horn.

The NAP project staff is particularly indebted to the following people:

Nursing students who assisted in bibliographic search and field testing

Marchita Butler	Edith Heideman
Susan Chou	Sr. Barbara Kennison
Debra Edwards	Cindy Leatherman
Sr. Barbara Gooding	Roberta Wetzel

Nursing service administrators in demonstration hospitals

Carolyn Cresswell	Eleanor Taylor
Judy Ivan	Orville Tews
Mary Morris	

Advisory Committee

Helen Berg	Mary Morris
Carol Boven	Eleanor Taylor
Marjorie Jackson	Orville Tews
Thelma Lauderbaugh	Laura Weng

This manual is the result of a project funded by the W. K. Kellogg Foundation in 1977–1978, and conducted at the Bureau of Hospital Administration, School of Public Health, University of Michigan, Ann Arbor.

PREFACE

This manual has been prepared to assist nursing service administrators in determining their current nursing assignment patterns and in making decisions regarding new patterns. While users will have their own ideas as to how this book can be utilized most profitably, it is our hope that readers will find the methodology informative and useful.

The manual provides the reader with the following:

Section I   Purpose of the Manual

Describes the rationale and assumptions of the approach.

Section II   Determining Your Assignment Patterns and and Directions for Change

Outlines a step-by-step approach to completing the four major phases of the process and reaching a data-based decision on the appropriate nursing assignment pattern for a patient unit.

Section III   Leadership Situations and Discussion Guide

Provides a method of introducing nursing personnel in leadership positions to the process.

Section IV   Instruments

Includes questionnaires required to collect data for determining nursing assignment patterns.

Section V   Coding Instructions

Provides instructions for handling collected data. Designed to help you understand and interpret your data so that meaningful analysis can be made.

Section VI   Connective Propositions

Links a unit's nursing assignment pattern with its patient characteristics, nursing resources, and organizational support. Contains guidelines for final decision making.

In organizing this manual we wish to integrate the material and provide continuity for the reader. The sections present, in orderly sequence, the process and a methodology for carrying it out.

TABLE OF CONTENTS

VII   Appendixes

LIST OF ILLUSTRATIONS

I

PURPOSE OF MANUAL

I

PURPOSE OF MANUAL

In spite of important differences in methods of delivering nursing care to hospital inpatients, there has been no ready way for nursing administrators to make careful and informed decisions about the most appropriate nursing assignment for their immediate situation. In part, this may be due to a tendency for scholars and some practitioners to focus on an ideal nursing process, and to de-emphasize the strong interdependence which nursing has with other parts of the hospital. This inevitably leads to a focus on which is the one best assignment pattern? rather than which assignment pattern will work best in this setting?

Recent work in the theory of organizations has provided support for a contingency model of organization, which replaces the "one best way" framework with one that recognizes the need to assess local conditions before deciding on the assignment pattern which is best for a given hospital unit, at a given time. The purpose of this manual is to provide a method of assessing local hospital conditions, to allow such informed decisions to be made.

Changing nursing assignment patterns is a major endeavor. If not done well it can result in failure to implement new patterns, increased dissatisfaction among nurses, and waste of time and money. Nursing, as the focal point for the delivery of inpatient care, needs an assessment tool to identify available and needed hospital and human resources. A plan for change can then be developed which involves obtaining needed resources and implementing reorganization in stages. This will increase the likelihood of a successful change and improve the quality of nursing care.

We have found it useful to go beyond the traditional nursing assignment patterns (functional, team, or primary) and to think of three major dimensions in any nurse utilization pattern. These three are:

1. The degree of division (or obversely, the integration) of nursing care given a patient; the elements are:
   Nursing Care Integration (NCI)
   Care Management Integration (CMI)
   Plan-Do Integration (PDI)
2. The degree of shifting (or obversely the continuity) of nursing personnel providing care for a patient; the elements are:
   Nursing Care Continuity (NCC)
   Care Management Continuity (CMC)
   Care Management Continuity across settings (CMCt)
3. The type of coordination used to plan and organize a patient's nursing care; coordination elements are:
   Nursing Coordination (NC)
   Care-Cure Coordination (CCC)
   Patient Services Coordination (PSC)
   Inter-Shift Coordination (ISC)

Figure I:1 gives the definitions we use for each of these elements. Because these definitions form the basis for the analysis of nursing assignment patterns, we suggest that you become familiar with them. The figure will also be a useful reference tool as you analyze the elements of current nursing assignment patterns.

The major variables which help determine the assignment pattern are: patient characteristics, nursing resources, and organizational support.

Data in these areas can provide the basis for evaluating your existing pattern and can suggest a direction for changing your pattern. Such data can also give you a basis for defending your present pattern. The specific data you will collect for these variables is presented in detail in Figures I:2, I:3, and I:4. Again, review these figures to familiarize yourself with them and use them as reference tools in your analysis.

Unless your hospital has the same kind of patients and staff in every unit, you should not expect to use the same assignment pattern on every unit. The organizational support for each patient unit will be similar (though not identical), and nursing resources will also have some similarities between units (though less than organizational support). The assessment tools provided in this manual are designed to help you study each patient unit separately to determine the assignment pattern needed. Specific data on the actual pattern in use provides a clear data base for planning modifications.

Of course, facts about your patient characteristics, nursing resources, and organizational support do not alone specify the best assignment pattern. These data must be organized into a usable format for analysis. In Section V, we provide detailed instructions for coding your data so that you can understand and analyze it. Your professional judgment can then be used to determine the most appropriate assignment pattern for the combination of patients, nursing resources, and support available for a patient unit.

Section VI of this manual presents a set of propositions connecting the major variables with different patterns. These propositions have been developed from an extensive literature review. Unfortunately, relatively little nursing research has aimed at improving nursing organization, and much of the literature consists of action reports rather than carefully designed research. Therefore, the connective propositions should not be a substitute for your professional judgment, but, rather, a framework within which your decisions will be made.

In addition to the above, you may wish to evaluate the results of any changes you implement. We provide explicit ways of measuring personnel satisfaction and more general directions for ensuring the availability of relevant cost data. Quality measures, though of major importance, are too complex to be included in this manual.

In summary, this manual is designed to show you how to gather data from your own hospital; how to analyze and compare them against published professional judgments and your own experience; and how to produce assignment pattern recommendations based on your supporting data. Such supporting data are crucial when cost pressures threaten the ability of nursing to deliver quality care. A data base also allows you to evaluate high-cost assignment patterns and encourages educated judgments regarding the best utilization of nursing personnel. This manual can be of help to you in determining your nursing assignment patterns and in deciding whether to keep or change those patterns.

Figure I:1
Elements of the Nursing Assignment Pattern

Variable Name		*Basis for Variable Definition*
Nursing Care Integration	NCI	The proportion of total care given by the person providing the most care.
Care Management Integration	CMI	The number of persons managing the care process at a given time.
Plan-Do Integration	PDI	The proportion of care givers also involved in the planning of care.
Nursing Care Continuity	NCC	The average number of care givers for a patient over a seven day period.
Care Management Continuity	CMC	The average number of care planners for a patient over a seven-day period.
Care Management Continuity across settings	CMCt	Whether a care planner is responsible for a patient before or after patient's stay on the unit.
Nursing Coordination	NC	An index which records the most common pattern of on-unit coordination of nursing care activities for a patient.
Care-Cure Coordination	CCC	Two indices which record the most common pattern of the nurse's direct involvement and the proactive-ness[1] of that involvement, in coordinating other
Patient Services Coordination	PSC	inputs to her patient's care requirements from physicians (CCC) and from other professionals (PSC).
Inter-Shift Coordination	ISC	An index which records the method of communication by which inter-shift coordination is achieved.

[1]proactive—taking the initiative in coordination activities, e.g., contacting other personnel, making referrals, problem-solving.
  reactive—not initiating; a passive or simply cooperative response to coordination initiatives from others.

Figure I:2
Patient Characteristics Variables

A. Age

Range: 0–99+ years
0–1   Infant
2–12   Child
13–20 Adolescent
21–65 Adult
66+   Elderly

The number of patients in the sample for each of five categories of age are tabulated from raw data on age in years.

B. Sex

Male or female.

C. Length of stay on unit

Range: 0–99+ days

Estimate of the entire duration of stay on the unit, for this admission only.

D. Instability[1]

Range: 1–15 points

Index of the degree of change in the patient's condition, based on degree of predictable change, condition class, and frequency of emergencies.

E. Variability[1]

Ranges:
a) Process 0–1.0 points
b) Therapy 0–1.0 points

The degree to which the sample patients are dissimilar (variable) in a) process requirements and b) therapy requirements.[2]

F. Uncertainty Factors:[1]

Indices of the degree to which patients' needs are not well understood.

    a) Predictability

Ranges:
Process 0–100%
Therapy 0–100%
Average 0–100%

The degree to which (at the time of data collection): a) nursing care requirements were predictable on the basis of the admitting medical description, and b) present and planned therapies were predictable on the basis of the initial medical work-up.

    b) Complexity of Processing[3]

Range: 0–100 points

The degree to which assessment, planning/or evaluation for nursing care are complex, in that a detailed history is required (1), multiple and complex problems are presented (5 and 6), feedback from patients (4) and problem solving (3) is necessary, and the nurses' initiative and work contribute to recovery (2).

    c) Complex Task Integration

Range: 0–1.0

The proportion of patients in the sample for whom integration of process and therapy tasks is complex, based on patient requirements in at least 8 different categories (4 process and 4 therapy).

G. Standardization

Range: 0–10 points

The degree to which standard care protocols or care plans are actually in use.

H. Multiple Technical
Requirements

Range: 0–1.0

The proportion of patients in the sample for whom difficult or multiple technical/mechanical therapies are in effect.

I. Multiple Learning Needs

Range: 0–1.0

The proportion of patients in the sample having substantial learning needs (at least three different areas of new learning).

J. Multiple Coordination
Needs

Range: 0–1.0

The proportion of patients in the sample having multiple (at least four) non-unit personnel involved in providing care.

---

[1]Based on Perrow's constructs (Perrow, Charles,"A Framework for the Comparative Analysis of Organizations," *American Sociological Review* 32 [3, April 1967]:194–208).

[2]Process requirements are common conditions or needs of clients requiring nursing knowledge and skills to assess, plan, intervene, and evaluate; therapy requirements are common therapies performed by or in collaboration with nursing personnel.

[3]Items are modifications of six items from the questionnaire presented in Overton, P., Hazlett, C. B., and Schneck, R., "An Empirical Study of the Technology of Nursing Subunits," *Administrative Science Quarterly* 22 (June 1977):203–19.

Figure I:3
Nursing Resources Variables

Variable		*Explanation*
Mix by Shift Ratio Day Evening Night	Ratio	Five-week average count of RNs/LPNs/Aides per shift transformed into a standardized ratio.
RN/Staff Ratio Day Evening Night	Ratio	Five-week average count of RNs/other staff per shift transformed into a standardized ratio.
RN/Patient Ratio	Ratio	Average number of patients per RN over a five-week period by shifts.
Part-time/Full-time Ratio	Ratio	Five-week average of part-time to full-time nursing personnel, all shifts.
Staff Commitment	Range: –6 to +6	Reasons for joining, staying, and leaving unit are assigned scores that reflect whether or not they are related to a commitment to patient care. Recorded separately for RN, LPN, Aides.
Staff Stability: a) Turnover	Range: 0–100%	Proportion of staff replaced each year, separately for RN, LPN, Aides.
b) Absenteeism	Range: 0–12%	Proportion of staff absent each day, separately for RN, LPN, Aides.
c) Staffing Instability	Range: 0–100%	The proportion of unit staff who change their unit or shift each day. Shown for RN, LPN and Aides separately for the day shift.
Staff Availability	No Range	An index of the labor market availability of different categories of nursing personnel.
Preparation Ratio	Ratio	The ratio of Master's + BSN, *To* Dip. + AD, *To* LPN + Aide in the total nursing staff on the unit.
Experience Ratio	Ratio	The average number of years of experience on the unit for Master's + BSN's *To* Dip. + AD *To* LPN + Aide.
Special Training	No Range	An estimate of the extent of special training, separately by RN, LPN and Aides, in five skill areas relevant to assignment pattern decisions.
In-Service Education Resource	No Range	A descriptive statement based on responses to questions about In-Service resources.

Figure I:4
Organizational Support Variables

Physician Presence	Range: 0–15	The amount of active physician presence on the unit, measured by the number of hours per week per patient that medical personnel are actively involved in care.
Physician-Nurse Communication	Range: 1–7	The formal systems of communication established in the areas of documentation, unit meetings, educational activities and patient rounds.
Physician-Nurse Collegiality	% Distribution	The physician's view of the nursing role as perceived by experienced nurses, ranging from subordinate role at the continuum's left to nurses as colleagues at the continuum's right.

Unit Support Services
  i Days-weekends
  ii Evenings-nights
Patient Care Support Services
  i Days-weekends
  ii Evenings-nights
	Range: 1–7
	
	Range: 1–7
		The amount of unit support and patient care services provided by personnel other than unit nursing staff, i.e. other hospital departments or other nursing department personnel. Also included in the score is the availability of coverage and the responsiveness to the nursing unit. The higher the score the more support services provided for unit and patient care activities and the better their responsiveness and availability.

Clinical Nurse Specialist Role	No Range	Specification of the major role played by the CNS.
Physical Environment	Range: 0–16	The proximity of the materials and communication systems to the patient room.
Financial Constraint	No Range	Descriptive statement of financial stringency based on three measures of hospital financial position.

II

DETERMINING YOUR ASSIGNMENT PATTERN AND DIRECTIONS FOR DECISIONS

II

DETERMINING YOUR ASSIGNMENT PATTERN AND DIRECTIONS FOR DECISIONS

Five major phases are important in determining your current assignment pattern and in deciding on an appropriate one:

A. preparing your organization
B. preparing yourselves
C. gathering data
D. coding and analysis of data
E. discussion and decision
F. evaluation

This manual does not deal with the final stage of implementing your decision, but it does include several actions intended to make implementation easier.

In this section, we provide a step-by-step outline for you and your Nursing Assignment Pattern (NAP) team to use in completing the four phases and reaching a data-based decision on the appropriate NAP for a patient unit.

The steps are intended as a guide to achieving certain definite results, which we summarize in a few sentences before each major set of steps. Keep the intended results foremost in your mind and skip or add steps as necessary to achieve those results. Assistance from someone who is experienced with this manual may be helpful. Steps where this might be particularly useful are marked with a (★).

A. Preparing your organization

Implement the principle of "never surprise people who have power."

1. Secure required organization approval for the analysis. The costs may include dollar outlays if you are using outside help, and will include time costs for you, your key people, and the nursing staff. You may want to bring the project to the medical staff executive committee's attention, in case you need support later on.

2. Select a group of 3–5 people who will be the team formally charged with the responsibility of collecting the data and

completing the NAP analysis. This team should be composed of people influential in determining nursing assignment patterns in your hospital.

This team will be involved in the implementation of whatever decisions are made based on the data collection and analysis. The success of the project may well depend on this team's effectiveness. Accordingly, the members should be given the status, recognition, and most important, the time to accomplish the task well. You will want to select a team name which best fits your hospital.

3. Send out a brief announcement to all nursing staff informing them of the study and the team. You may want to use part or all of the NAP Study Description found in Appendix 2.

B. Preparing yourselves

1. You and your selected NAP team should plan several sessions together. Independent completion of the "Leadership Situations" in Section III by all team members prior to the first group session will stimulate interest in assignment patterns. The discussion will also facilitate constructive clarification, sharing, and analysis of organizational values and goals. Begin using the concepts presented in Section I, such as nursing care integration, care management continuity, and other elements which make up the NAP conceptual framework.

2. The NAP team should become thoroughly familiar with Sections I and II of this manual. An additional information source is the article by F. C. Munson and J. Clinton, "Defining Nursing Assignment Patterns," in *Nursing Research* 28 (4, July-August 1979):243–49.

3. Members of the NAP team must develop the skills required for applying instruments in this manual prior to actual data collection. Training sessions will help the team collect reliable, valid, and complete data when on the study unit(s). We recommend skill practice sessions which specifically focus on each of the following tasks:

   a) After all NAP team members have had an opportunity to review the instru-

ments individually, conduct a group discussion on each instrument to share perceptions about commonalities and differences in how each of you interprets interviewer directions and/or directions to respondents who will be completing questionnaires. For example, areas which lead to disagreement could be recorded and posted on a blackboard or newsprint so that all can view them. The task then becomes one of deciding on a common way to manage these areas. Further exploration of the manual may be helpful in clarifying questions.

   b) A second session should be designed to brainstorm possible questions an interviewee may pose to data collectors, and to generate possible answers to give them based on group consensus and understanding of the manual's directions.

   c) One or more additional sessions should provide opportunities for skill practice in administering instruments in a learning environment. Each team member should have an opportunity to assume the role of data collector for instruments they will be administering. The purpose of these sessions should be to ensure that data collectors are collecting and recording data in a consistent manner. You will need some familiarity with coding instructions for each instrument (in Section V) to answer questions which will arise.

C. Gathering Data

Without a sufficient data base, no sound decision is possible. Be sure that you have a sense of *why* data is being collected, so that when questions come up about substitute data or interpretation, they can be handled informatively.

1. Identify the patient units that will be your initial study units. If you have a choice:

   a) Select more than one but fewer than five units. Comparison is useful, but too many units may make analysis difficult.

   b) Select units which are quite different from each other.

c) Select smoothly running units. Problem units can be handled more successfully in later analyses after you have had the opportunity to develop your study skills.

2. Identify nurse leaders on the unit; this may be only the head nurse or all the team leaders.

3. Meet with these leaders from all selected units to:

a) Describe study purpose and key variables. Prior to the meeting, it will be useful to hand out the NAP study description in Appendix 2.

b) Describe data collection requirements.

c) Set times and dates for training data collectors, for a test run using all instruments, and for the initiation of data collection.

★ 4. Collect Nursing Assignment Questionnaire and Patient Characteristics data (Section IV A & B).

a) Data will be collected on 5 patients in each administration of the questionnaires. Normally, the questionnaire will be administered three times, giving you a random sample of 15 patients. Space the data collection for each group of 5 patients about one week apart. If units have more than 40 patients, you will want to plan to collect data on more than 15 patients. In general, aim to collect data on 1/3 of your patient census plus about 5 patients. The following chart may be helpful.

Average Patient Census	1/3 Census	+5 =		Select a total patient sample of:
9	3	+5 =	8	(10)
21	7	+5 =	12	(15)
30	10	+5 =	15	(15)
42	14	+5 =	19	(20)
60	20	+5 =	25	(25)

b) Using a sample size different than 15 will require slight modifications when using coding instructions and reporting data on the display sheet.

c) Select a day of the week for data collection when staffing is typical.

d) Ensure that each sample is randomly drawn according to the procedure de-

scribed with the Nursing Assignment instrument. A random sample will give you sufficient data for the kind of analysis you need to do. It is neither necessary nor cost-effective to sample all patients.

e) A member of the NAP team should be selected to administer the Nursing Assignment and Patient Characteristics Questionnaires. This person should be present to assist the respondent the first time the questionnaires are completed. Unit nursing personnel should be encouraged to complete it on their own the second and third (or more) times.

f) Agree on who, beside the head nurse, will complete Question 26 of the Nursing Assignment Questionnaire.

5. Concurrently, arrange for completion of Data from Director and Nursing Office (Section IV E).

a) Make arrangements for having the appropriate persons complete each section.

b) Ensure that financial data is collected, and that, if necessary, alternative definitions of financial constraint are discussed and agreed on.

6. Concurrently, arrange for collection of Nursing Resources Questionnaire (Section IV C). Discussion with the head nurse should clarify exactly how the data will be accumulated for recording the weekly summaries.

7. Collect the Organizational Support data (Section IV D). Agree who besides the head nurse will be asked to complete page 3 of the questionnaire.

8. If you intend to use satisfaction data in your evaluation, arrange for anonymous completion by all RNs, and possibly LPNs, of the Staff Nurse Questionnaire (Section IV F). This instrument provides a baseline measure for personnel satisfaction for use in evaluation. Plan ahead for approval for use of the questionnaire, following your agency guidelines for use of human subjects. It is unwise to handle the analysis of this questionnaire internally. Therefore, arrangements for coding and analysis should be made in advance with an outside agency, so that all respondents may *know* that their re-

★ 9. Arrange for the collection or retrieval of unit cost data. There is no standard way to do this. Look at Collection of Cost Data (Section IV G), and determine the best way to secure baseline cost data for the study units.

    a) Collect or record baseline cost data for each study unit.

    b) Write out specific instructions so that exactly comparable data may be gathered at a later period.

  10. Determine the adequacy of your current measures of nursing quality. You may want to revise or add to these measures so that they will serve as a baseline measure of nursing quality for later use in evaluation.

D. Coding and Analysis of Data

At this point you have "mountains of facts, piled upon the plains of human ignorance." But it won't stay that way. Your next steps are to *review, code, display,* and *analyze* the data.

★ 1. Using the coding instructions, code all the Nursing Assignment Questionnaires for each unit. For *each* unit you should end up with a Nursing Assignment Display Sheet, an NCI graph, 2 worksheets, and pages 3, 4, 5 and 6. The key page is the Nursing Assignment Display Sheet; the other material is primarily supporting information that should be available for the analysis.

The coding of these data is time consuming, but do it carefully. Arithmetic errors can be very serious, either in leading to wrong conclusions, or in causing people to question the validity of your data.

★ 2. Using the coding instructions, code your Patient Characteristics data. Again you will have supporting data, but your key data summary will be on the Patient Characteristics Display Sheet.

  3. Complete the coding of your other data sources, using the same care you used for

the Nursing Assignment Display Sheet and the Patient Characteristics Display Sheet. Although these two will become central in the analysis, key constraints are often clarified in the Organizational Support and Nursing Resources Display Sheets.

4. Organize your baseline cost and quality data.

    a) Make sure whatever data you have decided to use for cost and quality measures are collected and the data stored in usable form, together with the data collection methods you used.

    b) File the analyzed satisfaction data from the staff nurse questionnaire, with the cost data and the quality data, and reserve them for later use in evaluation.

E. Discussion and Decision

This is the crucial stage, and the one at which the possibility of making changes as a result of the analysis begins to make future thinking about implementation important. At the end of this stage you should be able to affirm your present assignment pattern or decide on a better one. The steps below should help you reach this decision.

1. The NAP team should review all the digested data carefully, looking for inconsistencies or questionable data. The data should then be reviewed with unit leadership for the same purpose. Avoid combining this review with step 3 below; data verification *must* precede both your conclusions (step 2) and final decisions with unit leadership (step 3). You will sometimes find that unit personnel disagree with the data. For example, their patients are really more complex, more unstable, etc. They may be right. A sample of 15 patients taken over a three-week period does not ensure representativeness. On the other hand, perception that the data are inaccurate weakens the data's value, regardless of whether they are in fact accurate. If the personnel doubt the patient characteristics, you may need to take another sample. You will normally find that a second sample will turn up

some differences, which you can point to as supporting their doubts, but also that the basic characterization of the patient population will not change in a major way. When this is the case, several of the doubters will become supporters, and it will then be easier to deal with remaining doubts. Sometimes, just the willingness to repeat the work will get people thinking; they will begin to recognize that, for example, certain kinds of patients (difficult, challenging ones) tend to stand out, certain kinds of days (hectic, high-pressure ones) tend to be remembered, and that our judgments about the typical patient population are often colored by the more vivid memory of those kinds of patients and days.

The point is, be prepared to receive and deal with questions about your data base, to give these important people confidence in its accuracy.

★ 2. Using the Guide for Using Connective Propositions (Section VI A), and applying your own professional judgment and organizational knowledge, the NAP team should develop recommendations for modifying elements of the current pattern. Take this process element by element, thinking in terms of where you ought to be one or two years from now.
   a) Be explicit on the reasons for modifications, noting related key propositions or professional/organizational judgments.
   b) For each modification, note the expected result it will have in:
      • "pure" quality improvement;
      • quality improvement which will reduce length of stay (LOS);
      • "pure" cost improvement, direct reductions in payroll;
      • personnel satisfaction improvement, including those improvements which indirectly may improve costs. (reduced absenteeism, turnover, training costs, etc.)

★ 3. Give the recommendations to the leadership in each unit, and arrange for a discussion that will include an approval or modification of the recommendations, and a discussion of steps necessary to implement them. Such steps might include some of the following:

a) changing recruiting practices
b) encouraging medical staff to relate differently with nurses
c) changing the methods of admitting patients to units in order to reduce variability
d) training staff in documentation
e) adding staff to in-service training
f) developing ward clerk resources
g) developing better responsiveness in ancillary departments
h) discussing recommendations with affected collective bargaining organizations
i) changing physical facilities
j) special training in nursing process

★ 4. Work out a dated time-line specifying the steps to be undertaken. Estimate results, using the E2b categories above (or others, if preferable).

F. Evaluation

The evaluation step will be important both to you, in determining whether the change was a wise one, and to others when they assess the results of this investment of time and effort. The data requirements for evaluation have already been identified in B8, B9, and B10 of this section.

1. Develop an evaluation protocol that will allow inexpensive but reasonably accurate measures. Ensure that baseline data are complete, or can be readily retrieved from records at a later date. Note: Securing "proof" that a change in assignment pattern has had the intended results often costs more than it is worth. When five (or fifty) different things may influence costs, quality, or personnel satisfaction, designing and implementing an evaluation that shows the effects of a change of one of those five, or fifty, things is difficult and costly. We suggest that you take the shorter route of making sure you have reliable outcome data before and after the change and that you infer from internal evidence the extent to which differences in outcomes both before and after are to be attributed to the change being evaluated. Remember: scholars need to know causes, but practitioners need to get results.

2. Secure formal approvals of action to the extent required in your organization.
3. Because we intend to continue refining these nursing management tools, your evaluation of this manual, its usefulness and clarity, is needed. Appendix 5 details the three ways you can help us and to whom you can send your comments. Please take the time to write us a brief note; your feedback will be used.

Begin implementation. Good luck!

III

LEADERSHIP SITUATIONS AND DISCUSSION GUIDE

The ten leadership situations presented in this chapter should be responded to individually by nursing personnel in leadership positions (including at least yourself and all members of the NAP team), and then used to share and clarify values and goals in a group discussion. The discussions should lead into questions such as the following:

1. Is it important to have the responsibility for the care of a patient located in a single person?
2. What assignment pattern best suits the patient requiring multiple and complex care?
3. Is it appropriate to move toward different levels of care management integration, care management continuity or intershift continuity in your institution?

We have provided specific discussion questions for each situation to help your group get started, and they may help you think of other questions your group should address.

LEADERSHIP SITUATIONS AND DISCUSSION GUIDES

A. Situations

Below are several nursing unit or hospital situations. Depending on the organization, situation, and individual preferences of those involved, there may be several different appropriate goals in each situation, each one of them "good" in their particular context.

Please read each situation and write down the results or objectives you would want to achieve in handling the situation if it occurred in your organization. For the moment, ignore any constraints on the achievement of these objectives.

You may, as a good manager, be inclined to describe how you would handle this situation. DON'T. Write what you would *want to achieve*.

1. You hear good things from staff about a new head nurse on West Medical, and in talking with her you discover she has found a way to "... use the skills and interests of every member of the unit in direct patient service." The ward clerk handles dinner menu selection, one of the aides fills all water pitchers, one nurse (formerly with the VNA) handles discharge planning, another pours medications, etc. The head nurse herself is generally responsible for the care planning for all 20 patients.

Results or objectives you would want to achieve:

2. Several aides and an LPN from pediatrics have come to you with a complaint that they are being treated as unskilled servants rather than as members of a care team. "With this new primary business, the RNs think they own the patients. We don't even have team conferences any more. They think they're little doctors, with all their 'care plans' and 'nursing orders'. Why should they expect us to take an interest in patients when they treat us like we're not smart enough to think about patient needs?"

Results or objectives you would want to achieve:

3. "The third floor? Well, this morning Jane and Wilma both called in sick, and then Carol called and said there was some problem at the day school and she wouldn't be in. Pat and the other Carol both started vacation yesterday, and we had to pull from three different units before we got minimum safe coverage for the floor. And I'll bet we have 20 nurses mad, because they're caring for 'someone else's' patients and not 'their' patients. Hadn't we better give up pushing this idea of the same nurse caring for a patient from admission to discharge? It seems to me we're just making trouble for ourselves."

Results or objectives you would want to achieve:

4. Lots of complaints are coming from the RN staff about the use of written care plans. Some nurses say that since other nurses assess patients differently than they do, they have difficulty following the care plan prepared by nurses on another shift. So instead of cooperating with the care plan, some patients' care plans are actually being changed by nurses on each shift because of disagreements over the plan of care. The nursing staff wants to reduce the emphasis on care plans and instead expand shift reporting to 3/4-hour; they feel it is better for each nurse to plan the care of her patients herself, as long as every nurse knows, via shift reports, what the nurses on the other shifts are planning and doing.

Results or objectives you would want to achieve:

5. What you thought was a rather smooth-running application of progressive patient care in your hospital is being questioned by some of your new nurses. Recently they suggested that a single nurse be responsible for a patient from admission to discharge, doing all the care planning, teaching, discharge planning and even follow-up after discharge.

Results or objectives you would want to achieve:

6. You're turning over in your mind a rather strange incident that just took place. The head nurse on 2 West has just told you she *wants* AD nurses, doesn't want any more baccalaureates, and she's a baccalaureate herself. Apparently she has a style of management that gets everything tightly organized and lets all the problems come to her. She wants nurses that will fit in that structure, and apparently her experience is that four-year grads don't. You've had no complaints—in fact, the doctors praise her, say she's a crackerjack, etc. Of course the two four-year grads that were placed there dislike her intensely, and actually they're first-rate nurses.

Results or objectives you would want to achieve:

7. Another big fight. Mr. Phillips and his RN had planned together on rounds that he would receive instruction in wound care after breakfast and baths were finished. However, physical therapy had a cancellation at 9 a.m. and decided to take Mr. Phillips at 9 instead of 10. The result was

that his dressing was soaked by the time he returned to the unit, he was embarrassed about it, and also was too tired to participate in the dressing change. His nurse spoke to the physical therapy department, but they said they can't set up definite schedules because they have so many requests to fill—they just get as many done as they can. The nurse wants to know how she can get any discharge preparation finished if she can't plan ahead.
Results or objectives you would want to achieve:

8. During a departmental meeting, an argument develops about the proper use of four clinical nurse specialists (CNS) being hired next fall. One group wants each CNS made a part of a patient unit, to primarily provide care to highly acute patients in their specialty and thus to act as "role models" to staff. Another group wants to replace some head nurses, who will be retiring, with clinical specialists, so that their leadership will foster a stronger clinical focus and encourage the unit staff to develop their own expertise in giving and planning care. A third division disagrees completely, saying that all the clinical specialists should primarily act as expert consultants available to the whole nursing department, and be especially concerned with improving skills of staff nurses to deal with complex patients. One of the nurses present turns to you and says, "What do you honestly think is the best way to use them?"
Results or objectives you would want to achieve:

9. One of the younger nurses at Deaconess has become disturbed about the quality of the care planning on her unit. She has been called by several community agencies receiving patient referrals from her unit, about inaccurate information as to the patients' abilities and knowledge at discharge and their inability to carry out the nursing care as planned according to the referral. She wonders why this occurs, since the staff meet daily for brief team conferences, everyone contributes, and the team leaders and members all faithfully draft and revise the care plan as need arises, even though there are many other demands on everyone's time. She wonders if she should formally evaluate each nurse's care-planning abilities, or if the "team conference" system of planning is at fault.
Results or objectives you would want to achieve:

10. Interesting problem. Over the next three weeks you must prepare to fill certainly three, and maybe four, head nurse positions. Each of the four positions has a "natural" candidate, experienced, liked by the nurses and respected by the doctors; and not one of the four, when you come right down to it, is more than a good technical nurse. Minimal interest in patient teaching, even less in family teaching. The problem is that your staff nurses with a stronger professional orientation are less experienced, and apparently not interested in becoming head nurses.
Results or objectives you would want to achieve:

B. Discussion Guide for Leadership Situations

The purpose of the leadership situations given above is to open up a discussion. The following questions are addressed to each situation, and may prove useful in helping to focus the discussion on nursing assignment pattern issues. (We have found that some groups like to discuss their tactics as managers and avoid discussing what they want to achieve.)

Situation 1: Head nurse uses everyone. Issue: *Nursing Care Integration* (NCI).
1. Do some of you feel that ideally, all care for a patient should be done by one person? One team?
2. Do some of you feel that your preferences apply equally to all patients?

Situation 2: "RNs think they own the patients." Issue: *Care Management Integration* (CMI) and *Plan-Do Integration* (PDI).
1. How can LPNs and Aides best be used in patient care?
2. Do some of you feel that, ideally, both planning AND doing all the care for a patient should be done by one person? One team?

Situation 3: Nurses not caring for "their" patients. Issue: *Nursing Care Continuity* (NCC).
1. Is care continuity so important that strong efforts should be made to avoid changing patient assignments?
2. Do you feel this way for all patients?

Situation 4: Inter-shift problems with care plans. Issue: *Inter-Shift Coordination* (ISC).
1. What importance do you attach to:
   a) Having a single care plan guide the nursing care of all shifts?
   b) Having each shift accept full responsibility for patients?

Situation 5: Don't like progressive patient care. Issue: *Care Management Continuity* (CMC).
1. Do some of you feel that, ideally, one nurse should plan and manage the care of a patient from admission to discharge?
2. Does your feeling apply to all patients?

Situation 6: Head nurse who runs a tight ship. Issue: *Nursing Coordination* (NC).
1. Are there patient units where strong, directive leadership by a head nurse is desirable?
2. Ideally, do you want staff nurses to take full charge in managing the care of patients assigned to them?

Situation 7: Instructing a patient. Issue: *Patient Services Coordination* (PSC).
1. Ideally, how much do you want a nurse to be actively involved (proactive) in trying to get other departments to respond to her patient's needs?
2. Is it better for the head nurse to handle these outside department contacts?

Situation 8: Use of a clinical nurse specialist. Issue: *Clinical Nurse Specialist Role*.
1. What is the best way to utilize a clinical nurse specialist?
   a) As a role model and expert nurse for complex patient care?
   b) As a consultant and "back up" expert to train and assist staff in care?
   c) As an informal leader, with a focus on improving care and evaluation of quality?

Situation 9: Ineffective care planning. Issue: *Care Management Integration* (CMI).
1. Do some of you feel that effective care planning must be the responsibility of an individual?
2. Do some of you feel that, for some patients, preparing individualized care plans is a poor use of time?

Situation 10: Selecting head nurses. Issue: *Unit Leadership Requirements*.
1. How important is it to have a head nurse with a strong professional nursing orientation?
2. Will you need different skills and orientations in a head nurse if you change the nursing assignment pattern on a unit?

IV
INSTRUMENTS

This section includes the questionnaires required to collect data for determining appropriate nursing assignment patterns. As indicated on each form, the questionnaires are either self- or interviewer-administered instruments. We have provided specific instructions with each instrument. These instructions should be followed exactly. Note that the Nursing Assignment and Patient Characteristics Questionnaires will be administered more than one time depending on your unit size.

It is important that your NAP team adopt a consistent method for carrying out all data collection. This should include adequate time for checking rater reliability and a test run through the entire process before starting the actual study. In most hospitals it will require a minimum of two months to carry out this study and analysis.

Instruments for all parts of the data collection are included in this section. Sufficient copies for each unit will need to be copied from this manual. Do *not* use your original manual for data collection.

Remember, you are collecting data on the following key variables:

Nursing Assignment Pattern
Patient Characteristics
Nursing Resources
Organizational Support

A. NURSING ASSIGNMENT QUESTIONNAIRE

Directions to data collectors:

The data collected in this questionnaire will be used to describe the nursing assignment pattern currently in use on this unit. The questionnaire is designed to be used either by an interviewer, or to be self-administered. The questionnaire should be completed by the head nurse or the nurse(s) most qualified to describe current nursing assignment patterns on this unit. An NAP team member should be present to answer questions the first time this questionnaire is completed.

Special instructions are printed in CAPS. General instructions which apply to several parts of the questionnaire are given below. Read all instructions carefully, and refer to them when in doubt. Depending on the size of your unit, you will be administering the first part of the instrument (through Question 25) between one and three (or more) times. Space the data collections on each set of five patients about one week apart.

1. Use this opportunity to report conditions AS THEY ARE. DO NOT use it to prove how good they are, or how badly they need improving.
2. Student nurses: If student nurses are on your unit only 3–4 months a year or less, exclude patients who are being cared for by student nurses when drawing the sample. Otherwise leave them in.
3. Use "S" when reporting a student nurse.
4. Use "O" when reporting a non-unit person.
5. Write in clarifying comments when questions do not allow you to express the unit situation clearly.
6. Use a separate sheet of paper to keep track of patient names and numbers when you administer the first two questionnaires. To assure anonymity, it is important to NOT write the patients' names on the questionnaires. Be sure to destroy the sheet when you are done.
7. Reproduce two extra copies of Question 26 and attach them to the questionnaire before using.

IV A
Nursing Assignment Questionnaire

Unit _____   No. of Beds _____

Date _____   Head Nurse _____

Questionnaire
Administration # _____

In completing this questionnaire, the following items are needed:
 patient census for this unit:
 schedule for the past two weeks;
 nursing Kardex;
 today's assignment sheet;
 assignment sheets over the past week;
 patient charts.

Patient sample selection:
(1) Write the number of patients currently on the unit here: _____
(2) By any means, choose some number between 1 and the total number of patients. Write it here: _____
(3) Locate that number on the attached Random Number Table. (Use the 1–28 column, if the number of patients is 28 or less.) Record the next five numbers from the table that are less than or equal to the total number of patients (step 1). (DON'T INCLUDE THE NUMBER YOU CHOSE IN STEP 2 ABOVE.) _____
(4) Using the Kardex, patient census, or any other patient list, number the patients from one to whatever number of patients there are. (DON'T USE ROOM NUMBERS.)
(5) Identify the five patients who correspond to the five numbers chosen in step 3 above, and renumber these names from one to five on a sheet of paper. Keep this sheet by you throughout the Nursing Assignment and Patient Characteristic Questionnaires because the questions about these patients only refer to them by number. Do NOT write patient names or initials on the questionnaire, as this violates confidentiality. After you have filled out both questionnaires, destroy the sheet of paper with the names and numbers.

Record the diagnoses of the patients below.

	Major Diagnoses	Secondary Diagnoses
Pt. 1	_____	_____
Pt. 2	_____	_____
Pt. 3	_____	_____
Pt. 4	_____	_____
Pt. 5	_____	_____

Figure IV A:1
Random Number Table

Random Numbers 1–50		*Random Numbers 1–28*
30	43	09
21	37	11
01	08	01
18	20	06
29	42	18
19	31	25
11	35	10
39	04	12
34	28	04
25	17	19
03	24	07
27	26	22
14	46	13
12	32	05
07	22	15
05	41	08
36	47	03
16	06	20
45	44	28
13	38	17
48	50	02
49	40	26
23	02	23
15	09	16
10	33	27
		21
		24
		14

On this shift today, who would carry out each of these activities for the patients listed?

a) LEAVE BLANK THE ACTIVITIES WHICH WOULD NOT BE DONE TODAY.
b) WORK DOWN EACH COLUMN.
c) USE INITIALS TO IDENTIFY NURSING PERSONNEL DOING EACH TASK.
d) IF TWO NURSING PERSONNEL SHARE THE TASK TODAY, WRITE BOTH INITIALS.
e) IF STUDENT DOES TASK, WRITE "S".
f) IF NON-UNIT PERSONNEL DO TASK, WRITE "O".

NURSING CARE ACTIVITIES	PERSONS GIVING CARE TO:					CONTINUITY
	Pt.1	Pt.2	Pt.3	Pt.4	Pt.5	(Q 20–21)
1. Taking Temperature	/	/	/	/	/	
2. Taking Blood Pressure						
3. Taking Pulse and Respiration						
4. Assistance with Hygiene (routine bathing, skin and mouth care)						
5. Turning						
6. Range of Motion						
7. Administration of P.O. Meds						
8. Administration of I.M. Meds						
9. Administration of I.V. Meds						
10. Health Teaching for Patient and/or Family						
11. Recording Intake						
12. Recording Output						
13. Bed-making						
14. Treatments						
15. Assistance with Feeding						
16. Implementing Planned Assistance in Psychosocial Adjustment for Patient						
17. Implementing Planned Assistance in Psychosocial Adjustment for Family						
18. Preparation for Discharge						

Questions 19–22 refer to the Table above.

19. On this shift over a seven-day period, what is *the total number of different people* who
    would be taking temperatures:
        for patients such as patient 1?
        for patients such as patient 2?
        for patients such as patient 3?
        for patients such as patient 4?
        for patients such as patient 5?
    USE THE LOWER SEGMENT [⟍*] OF EACH BOX IN TEMPERATURE ROW
    TO RECORD ANSWER.
    REASONS FOR MORE THAN ONE CARE GIVER WILL BE RECORDED IN Q 22.

20. Record the most common response to Q 19 in the far right column of the Table, titled
    "CONTINUITY". If there is more than one common response, put both.

21. Record for the 17 remaining care activities the total number of people who would be
    doing each activity for the typical patient, over a seven-day period on this shift. Some
    activities are quite different from others, so look at each carefully. ENTER THIS
    NUMBER IN THE COLUMN MARKED "CONTINUITY."

22. Check the reasons below that more than one care giver per week is doing an activity for
    a patient.

Caused by regularly scheduled changes:	Caused by changes in patient needs:	Caused by changes in staff needs:
☐ days off	☐ change in care requirements	☐ caused by absenteeism/sickness, or need to float staff out
☐ shift rotation	☐ change in patient condition	
☐ assignment schedule	☐ heavy physical/ emotional demands of patient	☐ increase/decrease in census
☐ student rotations		☐ staff desire for variety
☐ other scheduled changes	☐ patient-staff conflict	☐ need for learning experience
	☐ other patient-induced changes	☐ staff desire to share work

NOW circle the 2 or 3 most important reasons you checked.

23. Now, consider the *management* of the care process (as distinct from who *gives* care) for the five patients chosen earlier. Who does each of the following activities for this shift today?

    a) USE INITIALS; WORK DOWN EACH COLUMN; LEAVE BLANK IF ACTIVITY NOT DONE.

    b) PUT ALL INITIALS IF TWO OR MORE PERSONS SHARE RESPONSIBILITY.

    c) INDICATE "S" FOR STUDENT, "O" FOR NON-UNIT PERSONNEL.

    d) IF PERSON WHO DOES CARE MANAGEMENT ACTIVITIES FOR THIS SHIFT IS ON ANOTHER SHIFT OR OFF TODAY, RECORD HER INITIALS AND EXPLAIN IN COMMENTS SECTION.

NURSING CARE MANAGEMENT ACTIVITIES	PERSONS MANAGING CARE FOR:				
	Pt.1	Pt.2	Pt.3	Pt.4	Pt.5
Securing Needed Patient Information					
Identifying Nursing Needs					
Stating Goals for Care					
Stating Interventions					
Evaluating Care					
Revising Interventions					

COMMENTS:

24. If the person or team you've identified in Q 23 will be responsible for all of the patient's care management during a seven-day period on this shift, put "1" in the box below for that patient. If not, put the number of persons or teams who will have responsibility during a seven-day period. Indicate with a "T," if the person or team you've identified in Q 23 will be responsible during patient's total stay on unit.

NO. OF PERSONS OR TEAMS
(specify which)
RESPONSIBLE DURING
7-DAY PERIOD

Pt.1	Pt.2	Pt.3	Pt.4	Pt.5

25. The following questions ask about the person/team you've identified in Q 23 as responsible for each patient's care management. Mark yes or no (Y or N) in the boxes for each patient.

The person/team you've identified in Q 23:

	Pt.1	Pt.2	Pt.3	Pt.4	Pt.5
Was responsible for patient prior to patient's transfer to this unit? (Leave blank if patient initially admitted to this unit.) (Y/N)					
Will be responsible for patient on transfer from this unit? (Leave blank if patient will be discharged from this unit.) (Y/N)					
Will be responsible for significant care management activities of patient after patient is discharged? (Y/N)					

STOP HERE IN THE SECOND AND THIRD ADMINISTRATION OF THE QUESTIONNAIRE.

Note: The questions which follow ask for an assessment of coordination practices on your unit. Select two other persons, possibly your immediate superior and your assistant head nurse, to fill out the second and third copies of these pages. Be sure the two persons you choose are knowledgeable about the four areas of coordination covered by the questions. Collect their responses and attach them to your questionnaire.

26. On the following chart (Figure IV A:2), we would like you to report coordination practices in four different areas, listed below:

Nursing coordination—This is coordination of the care activities for a patient performed by nursing personnel. The focus here is on the link between the person responsible for a patient and those who give the care.

Care-cure coordination—This is coordination between the patient's nurse(s) and the patient's physician(s).

Patient services coordination—This is coordination of the various patient activities (therapies, diet, tests, evaluation, etc.) done for a patient.

Inter-shift coordination—This is coordination from one shift to the next of the care activities performed by nursing and other personnel for a patient.

IN REPORTING COORDINATION PRACTICES, USE THE ALTERNATIVES SUGGESTED. USE SPACE BELOW FOR COMMENTS IF NEEDED.

COMMENTS:

Figure IV A:2
Coordination Practices Chart

	DEGREE OF ACTIVITY	FOCAL PERSON	METHOD	VEHICLE
	Degree of activity invested in this area of coordination. Think of the time spent to achieve it, the amount of training effort invested to have it done well, the attention given to follow-up or checking, how much coordination is emphasized as a key activity for one or more persons in this area. (Choose one) I-1 there is a major focus on achieving excellent coordination in this area I-2 we give quite a lot of attention to coordination in this area I-3 we try to ensure adequate coordination in this area I-4 a little effort is made in this area I-5 coordination is not really an issue in this area	Focal person who is primarily responsible for arranging coordination. Identify the person who, more than any other, accepts direct responsibility for this area of coordination. (Choose one) P-1 admitting physician P-2 intern or resident P-3 patient's nurse P-4 team leader P-5 head nurse P-6 other(s) (specify in box) P-7 no one	Method of achieving coordination. Identify the methods used by the focal person or by the organization to achieve coordination of this area. (Choose one) M-1 focal person does most activities directly, mainly coordinates own activities M-2 coordination achieved primarily by focal person actively collaborating with others in planning and care activities M-3 focal person less significant; coordination achieved primarily through persons following defined procedures M-4 coordination achieved primarily by focal person assigning or leading others	The vehicle or medium used to convey information in the coordination activity. (If more than one is significantly used, list the two most important.) V-1 integrated interdisciplinary care plans or progress notes, written specifically for individuals V-2 nursing care plans developed specifically for individuals V-3 oral report/or instructions V-4 discussion/conference V-5 informal conversations or phone calls V-6 standard care protocols/plans
Nursing Coordination	a	e	i	m
Care-Cure Coordination	b	f	j	n
Patient Services Coordination	c	g	k	o
Intershift Coordination	d	h	l	p

B. PATIENT CHARACTERISTICS QUESTIONNAIRE

Directions to data collectors:

The data collected in this questionnaire will be used to describe patient characteristics on this unit. The questionnaire should be completed by or with the nurse(s) most qualified to describe the patients and their needs. A NAP team member should be present to answer questions and clarify terms as necessary the first time this questionnaire is completed.

This questionnaire should be used in conjunction with the **Nursing Assignment Questionnaire.** Use the same patients you selected randomly for that interview. Major and secondary diagnoses for each patient are recorded on the Nursing Assignment Questionnaire. Refer to the sheet of numbered patient names from the previous questionnaire as you answer the questions here about Patient 1, Patient 2, etc. Destroy the sheet when the interview is completed. Remember that the patient numbers (1 through 5) should match the patient numbers identified in the **Nursing Assignment Questionnaire.** You should be using the same patients as those selected randomly for that questionnaire.

Before leaving the unit, check to make sure that the respondent followed the instructions under Question F.a. Predictability, to circle appropriate items on earlier pages of the questionnaire.

IV B
Patient Characteristics Questionnaire

Unit: _____   Date: _____

Respondent: _____   Questionnaire
                                 Administration #: _____

[USE SAME FIVE PATIENTS
AS IN PREVIOUS
QUESTIONNAIRE]

	Pt. 1	Pt. 2	Pt. 3	Pt. 4	Pt. 5
A. Age of patient Years:	____	____	____	____	____
B. Sex of patient (circle appropriate letter)	M F	M F	M F	M F	M F

C. Length of stay on unit

[RECORD NUMBER OF *DAYS*, NOT WEEKS]

	Pt. 1	Pt. 2	Pt. 3	Pt. 4	Pt. 5
1. Number of days since unit admission	____	____	____	____	____
2. Expected remaining length of stay on unit	____	____	____	____	____
Total	____	____	____	____	____

D. Instability

1. During the entire 24-hour day today, how often [are/were] the patient's vital signs or behavior likely to change? (If the patient will not be assigned continuously to *this unit* for all of today, consider *only the time he is assigned to this unit*.)

[CHECK APPROPRIATE BOX]

	Pt. 1	Pt. 2	Pt. 3	Pt. 4	Pt. 5
Less than once per day	☐	☐	☐	☐	☐
Twice per day	☐	☐	☐	☐	☐
Once per shift	☐	☐	☐	☐	☐
A few times per shift	☐	☐	☐	☐	☐
Every hour or more	☐	☐	☐	☐	☐

	Pt. 1	Pt. 2	Pt. 3	Pt. 4	Pt. 5

2. If the patient's condition (vital signs or behavior) deteriorated, would he probably remain on this unit?

	Pt. 1	Pt. 2	Pt. 3	Pt. 4	Pt. 5
Yes	[ ]	[ ]	[ ]	[ ]	[ ]
No	[ ]	[ ]	[ ]	[ ]	[ ]

3. Where and at what point on a scale of good/ fair/poor/serious/critical/dying, will or would the patient probably be transferred? If transfer would never occur, write "never".

Transfer to: When condition became good/fair/poor/serious/ critical/dying:

	Transfer to:	When condition became good/fair/poor/serious/critical/dying:
Patient 1	_____	_____
Patient 2	_____	_____
Patient 3	_____	_____
Patient 4	_____	_____
Patient 5	_____	_____

	Pt. 1	Pt. 2	Pt. 3	Pt. 4	Pt. 5

4. In general on this unit, how frequently do nursing personnel have to respond quickly to sudden changes in condition in patients such as this one?

	Pt. 1	Pt. 2	Pt. 3	Pt. 4	Pt. 5
Less than once a week	[ ]	[ ]	[ ]	[ ]	[ ]
About once a week	[ ]	[ ]	[ ]	[ ]	[ ]
Once every day or two	[ ]	[ ]	[ ]	[ ]	[ ]
About once every shift	[ ]	[ ]	[ ]	[ ]	[ ]
At least a few times per shift	[ ]	[ ]	[ ]	[ ]	[ ]

	Pt. 1	Pt. 2	Pt. 3	Pt. 4	Pt. 5

E. 1. Variability of Process Requirements

Which of the following conditions requiring nursing care does this patient have?

[IF CONDITION PRESENT, CHECK SPACE; IF NOT PRESENT, LEAVE SPACE BLANK. IF DON'T KNOW, WRITE IN "DK".]

Basic care conditions   *Row#*

	Pt. 1	Pt. 2	Pt. 3	Pt. 4	Pt. 5	Row#
immobility (partial or complete)	___	___	___	___	___	1
sensory deficit (numbness in hands or feet)	___	___	___	___	___	2
sight deficit	___	___	___	___	___	3
hearing deficit	___	___	___	___	___	4
speech deficit	___	___	___	___	___	5
incontinence (either bowel or bladder)	___	___	___	___	___	6
altered consciousness (disoriented or confused, obtunded, stuporous or comatose)	___	___	___	___	___	7
contagious or susceptible to infection (any type of isolation)	___	___	___	___	___	8
pain (any degree or type)	___	___	___	___	___	9
other (describe) _____ _____	___	___	___	___	___	10

Psychological needs

	Pt. 1	Pt. 2	Pt. 3	Pt. 4	Pt. 5	Row#
anxiety	___	___	___	___	___	1
depression	___	___	___	___	___	2
grieving	___	___	___	___	___	3
change in body image	___	___	___	___	___	4
dealing with impending death	___	___	___	___	___	5
other _____	___	___	___	___	___	6
other _____	___	___	___	___	___	7

	Pt. 1	Pt. 2	Pt. 3	Pt. 4	Pt. 5	

Social needs (patient or family)

"significant other" support (patient resources are reduced or absent; a moderate to large portion of support provided by staff) _____ _____ _____ _____ _____ 1

role adjustment (moderate to large) _____ _____ _____ _____ _____ 2

vocational adjustment (moderate to large) _____ _____ _____ _____ _____ 3

financial adjustment (moderate to large) _____ _____ _____ _____ _____ 4

environmental adjustment (moderate to large) _____ _____ _____ _____ _____ 5

Learning needs (patient and/or family)

new diagnosis _____ _____ _____ _____ _____ 1

new therapy _____ _____ _____ _____ _____ 2

new self-care _____ _____ _____ _____ _____ 3

new medications _____ _____ _____ _____ _____ 4

new diet _____ _____ _____ _____ _____ 5

modifications in activities of daily living or in lifestyle _____ _____ _____ _____ _____ 6

new means of communication (temporary or long-term) _____ _____ _____ _____ _____ 7

Spiritual needs

is requesting or in need of counsel _____ _____ _____ _____ _____ 1

Pt. 1   Pt. 2   Pt. 3   Pt. 4   Pt. 5

E. 2. Variability of Therapy
Requirements

Which of the following
diagnostic tests or
therapies are in effect now
or being planned for this
patient? (Other personnel
besides nursing staff may
be giving the care or
therapy.)

[IF TEST/THERAPY IS IN EFFECT
OR PLANNED, CHECK SPACE; IF NOT,
LEAVE SPACE BLANK.]

Basic care therapies   Row#

activity controlled (up
with assistance or
bedrest)   _____ _____ _____ _____ _____   1

stimulation controlled
(specified stimulation
either contraindicated
or required)   _____ _____ _____ _____ _____   2

hygiene assisted (set-up,
partial, or total bath)   _____ _____ _____ _____ _____   3

feeding assisted (set-up,
partial, or total feed)   _____ _____ _____ _____ _____   4

elimination assisted
(bathroom or commode
with help, or bedpan)   _____ _____ _____ _____ _____   5

Technical therapies

daily weights   _____ _____ _____ _____ _____   1

intake and output   _____ _____ _____ _____ _____   2

specimen collection   _____ _____ _____ _____ _____   3

vital signs   _____ _____ _____ _____ _____   4

wound/skin care (in-
cludes care of skin
around any drainage
sites or tubes)   _____ _____ _____ _____ _____   5

tube feeding   _____ _____ _____ _____ _____   6

intravenous therapy   _____ _____ _____ _____ _____   7

medications (all routes)   _____ _____ _____ _____ _____   8

	Pt. 1	Pt. 2	Pt. 3	Pt. 4	Pt. 5	

Technical therapies, continued

foley catheter	——	——	——	——	——	9
inhalation therapy (regular or prn)	——	——	——	——	——	10
physical therapy (e.g., range of motion, chest vibration, etc.)	——	——	——	——	——	11
other _____	——	——	——	——	——	12

Mechanical therapies

monitor and/or respirator	——	——	——	——	——	1
chest suction	——	——	——	——	——	2
nasogastric suction	——	——	——	——	——	3
tracheostomy (new or old)	——	——	——	——	——	4
other suction	——	——	——	——	——	5
dialysis (hemodialysis or peritoneal dialysis)	——	——	——	——	——	6
stryker frame (with or without traction)	——	——	——	——	——	7
traction (any type)	——	——	——	——	——	8
other _____	——	——	——	——	——	9

Observational requirements

[CHECK ONLY ONE; IF NONE, LEAVE BLANK]

routine	——	——	——	——	——	1
observe at 2–4 hour intervals, being alert for possible changes	——	——	——	——	——	2
observe frequently, about every hour	——	——	——	——	——	3
observe every half hour or more	——	——	——	——	——	4

| | Pt. 1 | Pt. 2 | Pt. 3 | Pt. 4 | Pt. 5 | |

Patient care services

[IF SERVICE IS IN EFFECT
OR PLANNED FOR PATIENT,
CHECK BLANK; IF NOT,
LEAVE SPACE BLANK]

	Pt. 1	Pt. 2	Pt. 3	Pt. 4	Pt. 5	
diagnostic tests	___	___	___	___	___	1
medication instruction (by pharmacist)	___	___	___	___	___	2
diet instruction (by dietician)	___	___	___	___	___	3
inhalation therapy (by therapist)	___	___	___	___	___	4
physical therapy (by therapist)	___	___	___	___	___	5
occupational therapy (by therapist)	___	___	___	___	___	6
home care or placement planning (with a department or agency)	___	___	___	___	___	7
consultation with:						
medical specialist(s)	___	___	___	___	___	8
nursing specialist(s)	___	___	___	___	___	9
social worker	___	___	___	___	___	10
clergy	___	___	___	___	___	11
other _____	___	___	___	___	___	12
patient care staff involved with this patient:						
attending physician	___	___	___	___	___	13
resident(s)	___	___	___	___	___	14
interns and/or medical students	___	___	___	___	___	15
nursing students	___	___	___	___	___	16

Pt. 1 Pt. 2 Pt. 3 Pt. 4 Pt. 5

F. Uncertainty

a) *Predictability*

1. Go back to item E.1. and *circle* the √s or Xs of those *nursing needs or problems* which were predictable for this patient on the basis of his *admitting medical description.*

[CODER: Calculate and record the percentage that was predictable.

____% ____% ____% ____% ____%

2. Go back to item E.2. and *circle* the √s or Xs of those *tests or therapies* which were predictable for this patient *after the initial medical workup.*

____% ____% ____% ____% ____%]

b) *Complexity of processing*

1. For this patient, how important is it to know a detailed history from birth to present in order to plan his/her care?

[CHECK APPROPRIATE BOX]

	Pt. 1	Pt. 2	Pt. 3	Pt. 4	Pt. 5
very high importance	☐	☐	☐	☐	☐
high	☐	☐	☐	☐	☐
moderate	☐	☐	☐	☐	☐
fair	☐	☐	☐	☐	☐
little or no importance	☐	☐	☐	☐	☐

2. What percentage of the time does improvement in this patient's condition really depend upon the skillful work and initiative of nursing personnel?

	Pt. 1	Pt. 2	Pt. 3	Pt. 4	Pt. 5
100%	☐	☐	☐	☐	☐
75	☐	☐	☐	☐	☐
50	☐	☐	☐	☐	☐
25	☐	☐	☐	☐	☐
0	☐	☐	☐	☐	☐

3. What percentage of this patient's nursing care relies upon nurses' problem-solving rather than on set procedures or routines?

	Pt. 1	Pt. 2	Pt. 3	Pt. 4	Pt. 5
100%	☐	☐	☐	☐	☐
75	☐	☐	☐	☐	☐
50	☐	☐	☐	☐	☐
25	☐	☐	☐	☐	☐
0	☐	☐	☐	☐	☐

4. How much of the patient's care plan changes in direct response to changes in the patient's condition or mood?

	Pt. 1	Pt. 2	Pt. 3	Pt. 4	Pt. 5
100%	☐	☐	☐	☐	☐
75	☐	☐	☐	☐	☐
50	☐	☐	☐	☐	☐
25	☐	☐	☐	☐	☐
0	☐	☐	☐	☐	☐

5. Some patients have one main health problem; others have several interrelated health problems. How many *health problems* does this patient have?

[RECORD # HEALTH PROBLEMS]

____ ____ ____ ____ ____

6. In terms of the total care planning, does this patient have *complex* problems that are not well understood? How many of these kinds of complex problems does he/she have?

[RECORD # COMPLEX PROBLEMS; IF NONE, RECORD 0]

____ ____ ____ ____ ____

Pt. 1   Pt. 2   Pt. 3   Pt. 4   Pt. 5

G. Standardization

[CHECK APPROPRIATE BOX]

For those aspects of medical and nursing
care which were predictable when the patient
was admitted to the unit, are standardized
protocols or care plans being used?

	Pt. 1	Pt. 2	Pt. 3	Pt. 4	Pt. 5
yes, for all aspects	☐	☐	☐	☐	☐
yes, for most aspects	☐	☐	☐	☐	☐
yes, for many aspects	☐	☐	☐	☐	☐
yes, for some aspects	☐	☐	☐	☐	☐
yes, for few aspects	☐	☐	☐	☐	☐
no, nothing standardized	☐	☐	☐	☐	☐

END OF QUESTIONNAIRE

THANK YOU.

Figure IV B:1
Patient Characteristics Questionnaire Worksheet

This worksheet allows the coder to tabulate the variables of *complex task integration* and *multiple technical, learning, and coordination requirements*. It should be attached to each ques-tionnaire. The coder should follow the instructions below. The rest of the Worksheet will be filled out later when coding the entire questionnaire. See the Patient Characteristics Coding Instructions (pp. 81–93).

CODER: Record the *number of items checked* within each category of requirements (pp. 3–7). Do *not* include "don't know" items!

E.1 Process Requirements: Pt. 1 Pt. 2 Pt. 3 Pt. 4 Pt. 5

  Basic care conditions ____ ____ ____ ____ ____

  Psychological needs ____ ____ ____ ____ ____

  Social needs ____ ____ ____ ____ ____

  Spiritual needs ____ ____ ____ ____ ____

  Learning needs ____ ____ ____ ____ ____ → _____
                                                               Multiple
                                                       Learning Needs

      (√) ____ ____ ____ ____ ____
              Complex process integration

E.2 Therapy Requirements:

  Basic care therapies ____ ____ ____ ____ ____

  Technical therapies ____ ____ ____ ____ ____

  Mechanical therapies ____ ____ ____ ____ ____
    check if patient has:
    monitor or
    respirator or (√) ____ ____ ____ ____ ____
    hemodialysis or
    peritoneal dialysis or
    stryker frame or
    new tracheostomy → _____
                                                              Multiple
                                                          Technical
  Observational   Requirements
  requirements ____ ____ ____ ____ ____

  Patient care services ____ ____ ____ ____ ____ → _____
                                                          Multiple
                                                           Coordination
      (√) ____ ____ ____ ____ ____   Needs
            Complex therapy integration

      (√) ____ ____ ____ ____ ____ → _____
          Complex process *and* therapy   Total
                    integration   Complex Task
                                                           Integration

C. NURSING RESOURCES QUESTIONNAIRE

Directions to data collectors:

The data collected in this questionnaire will be used to describe the nursing resources on this unit. The questionnaire should be completed by or with the head nurse. Note that the data is collected over a period of five weeks in order to (1) obtain average scores for available nursing personnel per shift* and (2) determine rotation/flotation patterns.

It is important to collect this data for all levels of nursing personnel including RNs, LPNs, and aides. Specific instructions for this data collection are included with the first two pages of the questionnaire.

We have not included an instrument for measuring staff commitment, although commitment is a significant variable recognized in the literature as an important influence on the success of nursing assignment patterns. We suggest that, rather than seeking data on this difficult to measure and sensitive variable, you use absenteeism as a proxy measure, modified by your own judgment about the level of commitment in the unit's nursing staff.

---

*If you intend to use data ONLY FROM A SINGLE SHIFT, collect data for that shift only. Be sure to instruct data gatherers and respondents accordingly.

IV C
Nursing Resources Questionnaire

Unit _____

Dates: from _____ to _____

Staffing Record

Over the next five weeks, keep a record of (1) the number (by category) of different nursing personnel on your unit for each shift every day, (2) the number of people absent in each personnel category per day, and (3) the daily patient census. At the end of each week, calculate and record below: (1) the *average* daily number of personnel in each category for each shift that week, (2) the *average* daily absenteeism in each personnel category that week, and (3) the *average* daily patient census for the unit that week. Include both weekdays and weekends in your calculations. It is important that you select a five-week period that does not include major holidays or vacations. If such a week would be included, don't use it but collect data on the next regular week instead.

Check with those arranging the data collection to see if data for all shifts are required.

AVERAGE NUMBER OF NURSING PERSONNEL PER SHIFT BY LEVELS AND AVERAGE PATIENT CENSUS FOR WEEKS 1-5

	Week #1	Week #2	Week #3	Week #4	Week #5	5-Week Average
Average number of RNs/shift:						
Days						
Evenings						
Nights						
Average number of RNs Absent/day:						
Average number of LPNs/shift:						
Days						
Evenings						
Nights						
Average number of LPNs Absent/day:						
Average number of Aides/shift:						
Days						
Evenings						
Nights						
Average number of Aides Absent/day:						
Average Daily Census:						

Staffing Instability and the Rotation/Flotation Record

For the same five weeks, keep a daily record of (1) the number of people in each personnel category who floated onto your unit during the day shift, (2) the number of people in each personnel category who floated off your unit during the day shift, (3) the number of people in each personnel category who rotated to/from the evening shift to/from the day shift (that is, between these shifts), and (4) the number of people in each personnel category who rotated to/from the night shift to/from the day shift (that is, between these shifts).

At the end of each week, *record the average score* for the above four items in the table below.

AVERAGE ROTATION AND FLOTATION SCORES
FOR FIVE-WEEK PERIOD BY LEVEL OF PERSONNEL

	Wk. #1	Wk. #2	Wk. #3	Wk. #4	Wk. #5
Data for RNs:					
1) Average number of RNs floating onto unit during day shift					
2) Average number of RNs floating off unit during day shift					
3) Average number of RNs rotating to/from evening shift to/from day shift.					
4) Average number of RNs rotating to/from night shift to/from day shift.					
Data for LPNs:					
5) Average number of LPNs floating onto unit during day shift.					
6) Average number of LPNs floating off unit during day shift.					
7) Average number of LPNs rotating to/from evening shift to/from day shift.					
8) Average number of LPNs rotating to/from night shift to/from day shift.					
Data for Aides:					
9) Average number of Aides floating onto unit during day shift.					
10) Average number of Aides floating off unit during day shift.					
11) Average number of Aides rotating to/from evening shift to/from day shift.					
12) Average number of Aides rotating to/from night shift to/from day shift.					

Special Training

In the table below, *estimate* the percent of staff personnel who have had special training, beyond basic education, since joining your unit in the areas listed on the left of the table. Exclude basic orientation training unless it includes the content areas listed. Completion of the table *does not require exact* answers but only estimates. If you are unsure of your estimates perhaps you might consult with inservice personnel to supplement your own judgment.

Record the percent of your total staff who have had the training *above* the diagonal line in each box.

	RN		LPN		Aides	
	%	hrs.	%	hrs.	%	hrs.
a) Documentation in charting (e.g., problem-oriented or other charting system)						
b) Use of nursing process						
c) Leadership and interpersonal skills						
d) Training intended to facilitate individual accountability						
e) Medications						

Approximately how many hours are spent training each person in each personnel category and area you marked? Record the typical number of hours spent training each person *below* the diagonal line in each box.

D. ORGANIZATIONAL SUPPORT QUESTIONNAIRE

Directions to data collectors:

The data collected in this questionnaire will be used to describe the organizational support on this unit, such as medical personnel, unit support services, patient care support services, and general environmental support services. The questionnaire should be completed by or with the head nurse.

It is important to read through the entire questionnaire before starting and to note the order for completing the columns of the support services question. Column I should be completed before going on to Column II and III.*

Reproduce two extra copies of the Physician-Nurse Collegiality questions under A 3.1-3.3 (page 3 of questionnaire).

---

*If you intend to use data ONLY FROM A SINGLE SHIFT, collect data only from that shift. Be sure to instruct data gatherers and respondents accordingly.

IV D
D. Organizational Support Questionnaire

Unit _____

Date _____

A. Medical Resources

1. Active physical presence of medical personnel on this unit.

	Total hours per week members of group spend giving care on unit. Exclude hours of on-call availability; count only hours of active presence.
Private physicians (attending, specialists, consultants)	_____
Fellows	_____
Residents	_____
Interns	_____
Physician assistants	_____
Medical students	_____
Total number of hours for all groups	_____

2. What are the predominant systems of communication between physicians and nurses? Mark the appropriate boxes to describe the systems used.

    2.1 Rounds with doctors:

        Regularly used   ☐ ⟶

        Irregular or none (Go to Question 2.2) ☐

> Nurse primarily collaborates with MD on care plan. ☐
>
> Doctor primarily informs nurse of care plan. ☐

    2.2 Scheduled joint educational sessions:

        Regularly used   ☐ ⟶

        Irregular or none (Go to Question 2.3) ☐

> Usually a discussion between nurses and physicians. ☐
>
> Usually lecture by physician ☐
>
> Usually lecture by nurse ☐

    2.3 Meetings on the unit:

        Regularly used   ☐ ⟶

        Irregular or none (Go to Question 2.4) ☐

> Usually collaborative discussion of patient care between nurse and physician. ☐
>
> Usually physician provides information to nurse. ☐
>
> Usually nurse provides information to physician. ☐

    2.4 Integrated medical record (all health professionals contribute to same progress notes and/or problem list):

        Yes   ☐   No   ☐

Note: The following questions ask for an assessment of physician perceptions of the nurses' role. Select two other persons, possibly your immediate superior and your assistant head nurse, to fill out the second and third copies. Be sure the two persons you choose are knowledgeable about the medical staff active on your unit. Collect their responses and attach them to your questionnaire.

3. Physician-Nurse Collegiality

The three following questions seek an estimate of physicians' perceptions of the nursing role. Note in each box below the percent of the unit's physicians who perceive nurses' role in this manner. Remember to check that each scale's percentages add up to 100%.

3.1 Independent functions:

%	%	%	% = 100%
Physicians recognize only dependent functions as the true nursing role.	Physicians view dependent functions as the primary nurse role.	Physicians recognize independent functions as occasionally important to patient care.	Physicians view independent nursing functions as the primary nurse role.

3.2 Doctor-nurse coordination:

%	%	%	% = 100%
Physicians expect nurses to only follow orders.	Physicians expect nurses to follow orders and provide relevant information.	Physicians expect nurses to be junior colleagues in some care management decisions.	Physicians view nurses as the expert member of care team for certain care management activities.

3.3 Stereotyping:

%	%	%	% = 100%
Physicians view all nursing staff as narrowly trained semi-professionals.	Physicians distinguish only between nurses and aides, and rely on familiarity with staff to distinguish ability of nurses.	Physicians recognize differences within the RN group, but are unclear on distinctions related to professional preparation.	Physicians understand and have different expectations of differently trained RNs.

B. Support Services

This question is concerned with the source, availability and responsiveness of support services to nursing needs. Listed below are a variety of support services required for patient care. In the first column, indicate the department responsible for providing the service, using the symbols at the top of the column. If two groups provide significant amounts of the same service, put both letters in the column. Move down the first column, then read the instructions at the end of the table before completing Columns II and III.

	I Responsibility for Providing Service U=Unit nursing (RNs, LPNs, Aides) O=Other nursing dept. personnel H=Other hospital departments X=Not used	II Absence of Coverage Place √ only if services are both unavailable and needed				III Responsiveness to Nursing Needs G=Good F=Fair P=Poor
		Day	Wknd	Eves	Nite	
1. Unit Support Services a. Technical: Specimen collection						
Patient transportation						
Messenger service						
Ordering and stocking supplies						
Laundry stocking & disposal						
Unit housekeeping						
Unit maintenance						
b. Clerical: Unit records						
Scheduling patients & appointments						
Phone answering						
Transcribing MDs orders						
Processing unit admissions						
Processing unit discharges						
Receptionist duties						
c. Administrative: Recruitment						
Staff scheduling						
Arranging daily coverage						
Patient classification						
New nurse orientation						
Staff education						
Other unit support of administrative functions						

	I Responsibility for Providing Service	II Absence of Coverage				III Responsiveness to Nursing Needs
	U=Unit nursing (RNs, LPNs, Aides) O=Other nursing dept. personnel H=Other hospital departments X=Not used	Place √ only if services are both unavailable and needed				G=Good F=Fair P=Poor
2. Patient Care Support Services		Day	Wknd	Eves	Nite	
a. Medications: Use of unit dose						
Medication distribution						
Floor pharmacist						
Discharge teaching						
b. I.V. Therapy: Mixing I.V.s						
Handling I.V.s						
Inserting I.V.s						
c. Diet: Food service to patients						
Menu selection assistance						
System for altering diets						
Diet teaching						
Feeding patients						
d. Social Support: Discharge planning						
Family counseling						
Housing arrangements						
Psychological counseling						
Referrals to outside agencies						
Coordination of planning with family						
e. Patient Education:						
f. Physical Therapy:						
g. Occupational Therapy:						
h. Speech Therapy:						
i. Inhalation Therapy:						
j. Nurse Specialists:*						
k. Other Patient Services; specify which, below:						

*Note below whether the primary role of the nurse specialist is staff development, patient care, or consultation.

READ THE INSTRUCTIONS ON THE NEXT PAGE BEFORE GOING BACK TO COLUMNS II AND III

DO NOT COMPLETE "ABSENCE OF COVERAGE" AND "RESPONSIVENESS" COLUMNS OF QUESTION B, IF AN "X" APPEARS IN THE FIRST COLUMN.

Some of these support services may not be needed on days, evenings, and nights. Others may be needed but not available. Go back to the second column (Absence of Coverage) and place a check [√] only in the boxes where coverage is both needed and unavailable. Check with staff on other shifts if you are uncertain about the availability of coverage on other shifts. In the third column, rate the Responsiveness to Nursing Needs for each service. Responsiveness is defined as the promptness, efficiency and readiness to respond to patient or nursing needs. Generalize for all affected shifts in judging this. Use a "G" if the service is good in its responsiveness to needs, an "F" if the service is fair, and a "P" if the service is Poor.

C. Physical Environment

    1. Proximity of materials (indicate location of the following; check *one* in each row):

	Patient Rooms	Near All Rooms	Mobile Carts	Central Location But Far From Some Rooms
Clean Linen	_____	_____	_____	_____
Central Service Supplies	_____	_____	_____	_____
Medical Records	_____	_____	_____	_____
Medications	_____	_____	_____	_____
Waste Disposal	_____	_____	_____	_____
Linen Disposal	_____	_____	_____	_____

    2. Communication system (check appropriate column):

	Yes	No
Telephone in or near patient's room for nurse use	_____	_____
Pocket pager	_____	_____
Intercom and call light from patient's room to nursing station	_____	_____
Nurse call light only	_____	_____

Comments:

E. DATA FROM DIRECTOR AND NURSING OFFICE

Directions to data collectors:

The data collected in this section will be used to supplement the data on Nursing Resources and Organizational Support you have already collected. You may need to collect this additional data from several sources, possibly including the Director of Nursing, the Personnel Office, and the Chief Financial Officer.

This instrument will provide specific information regarding:

A. Nursing resources
    Unit staff data
    Staff availability
    Unit staff turnover
    In-service assessment
B. Organizational support
    Financial constraints

IV E
Data from Director and Nursing Office

Unit _____

Date _____

A. Nursing Resources

Unit Staff Data

Write in names of all full-time and part-time RNs, LPNs, and aides currently employed on this unit. Place a check in the appropriate columns beside each staff name. Precise data is not necessary for years of experience. Place "HN" in front of name of head nurse, and "AHN" in front of name(s) of assistant head nurses, if any.

Name	Nursing Education				Years of Experience on Unit					Part-time (P) Full-time (F)	
	MSN, BSN	AD, Dip.	LPN	None	1 or less	2	3	4	5+	P	F

Staff Availability

Indicate below the level of availability of various types of nursing personnel. Place a check in the appropriate column.

	Scarce, Difficult to Recruit	Available	Ample, Applicants Waiting for Employment
RN: BSN			
RN: AD			
RN: Dip.			
LPN			
Aides			

Unit Staff Turnover

Record the number of new hires, transfers to and from the unit, and terminations for each personnel category on this unit over the past 6 months. Include part-time personnel.

Period covered: From _____ to _____ .

	New hires to this unit	Transfers *to* this unit	Transfers *from* this unit	Terminations from this unit
RNs				
LPNs				
Aides				

In-Service Assessment

A part of the data requirement for the NAP analysis is an assessment of the in-service educational resource. We suggest that three knowledgeable persons answer the questions below, and by comparing their answers reach a joint assessment. Check the box that most appropriately describes the *quality* of various aspects of the resource.

	Poor	Fair	Good	Excellent
a) The *technical* competence of either in-service staff or resource people (e.g., clinicians) to provide advanced, specialized clinical training.	☐	☐	☐	☐
b) The teaching competence of both in-service staff and resource people to communicate clearly.	☐	☐	☐	☐
c) Evaluation of performance following in-service programs.	☐	☐	☐	☐
d) Adequacy of budget support for release time for attending in-service and continuing education programs.	☐	☐	☐	☐
e) The space, equipment and facilities needed for training.	☐	☐	☐	☐
f) Funds and arrangements which allow nurses to attend training opportunities outside the hospital.	☐	☐	☐	☐
g) The hospital's ability to provide orientation for new and inexperienced nurses.	☐	☐	☐	☐

General Comments:

_____

_____

_____

_____

B. Organizational Support

This information may be most easily secured from the hospital's chief financial officer.

Financial Constraint

1. Margin of hospital net revenues over expenses (or under; specify which):

    Two fiscal years ago (percent)   ————

    Last fiscal year (percent)   ————

    Current fiscal year budget (percent)   ————

2. Proportion of net revenues received from 3rd party payers:

    Last fiscal year   ————

3. Hospital occupancy (percent):

    Two fiscal years ago   ————

    Last fiscal year   ————

    Current year to date   ————

F. STAFF NURSE QUESTIONNAIRE

Directions to data collectors:

The data collected in this questionnaire will provide a baseline measure of staff nurse satisfaction. The questionnaire should be completed by individual staff nurses. Approval to carry out this part of the study must be obtained from your hospital Human Subjects Review Committee prior to seeking participation by staff nurses.

An explanation of the study and the projected use of the data must be given to all participants prior to their completion of the questionnaire. They must be informed that they have the right to answer all or part of the questions and the right to refuse to participate. Avoid collecting and analyzing this data yourself *if at all possible*. If you cannot, the first two questions should be eliminated. Anonymity must be assured and nurses should *not* sign these questionnaires. Use the following procedure in administering the instrument:

(a) Use the "Unit Staff Data" from the previous questionnaire to identify the names of persons to receive this questionnaire.

(b) LPNs should be included if they play a significant role in patient care.

(c) Note that no data from this questionnaire should be analyzed unless there are at least four respondents in each category you wish to analyze, e.g., total staff or RNs or LPNs or Aides.

(d) Include sealable envelopes, properly addressed and stamped if necessary, with every questionnaire.

IV F
Staff Nurse Questionnaire

We are asking you to participate, along with many other nursing personnel in this hospital, in a survey being conducted for us by [insert name of organization conducting the survey] .... We hope you will agree to complete this questionnaire, and return it in the enclosed envelope. Your responses will be kept strictly confidential, particularly as far as any one in the hospital is concerned.

This survey is part of a study which is directed toward evaluating our nursing assignment patterns. We are interested in how patient units are organized and how the work of each unit is carried out. Your responses to this questionnaire will give us valuable baseline information on the satisfaction of nursing personnel, and the entire study should produce significant information concerning patterns of organizing the patient care team.

Thank you very much.

Unit _____

Date _____

Background Information

1) How long have you worked on your present unit? (check one)

    1. [ ] Under a year

       [ ] A year or more

2) What is your education in nursing?

_____

Job Characteristics

In the following questions we would like you to give an objective appraisal of the opportunities for satisfaction in your nursing work.

Listed below are 10 characteristics connected with your work, such as the opportunity to share in decisions, to work closely with likeable people, etc. Each characteristic will be followed by questions (a) and (b).

We use a seven-point scale to let you express differences in your feelings about the questions. *Circle the number* that represents how much of the characteristic being rated (a) *is* and (b) *should be* in your job.

Low numbers represent low amounts and high numbers represent high or maximum amounts. If you think there is "very little" or "none" of the characteristic associated with your job, you would circle number 1. If you think there is "just a little," you would circle number 2, and so on. If you think there is a "great deal but not a maximum amount," you would circle number 6. For each scale, *circle only one number.*

Please do not omit any scales.

An example is presented below. The question was answered by a nurse and her later comments about it are included to help clarify the nature of the questions. NOTE: You should NOT write explanations on your own questionnaire.

The *opportunity to fully use my skills and abilities* in my job:

a. How much is there now?   [none at all] 1 2 3 4 5 6 7 [maximum]

(We have had poor support personnel; I am doing aide's work.)

b. How much should there be?   [none at all] 1 2 3 4 5 6 7 [maximum]

(There is need to reorganize the work more, though in this job all of my skills and abilities can never be fully used.)

Note that in (b), "How much should there be?" you are evaluating your position in terms of how much it *could* provide of the characteristic in question.

1. The *opportunity to fully use my skills and abilities* in my hospital job:

   a. How much is there now?   [none at all] 1 2 3 4 5 6 7 [maximum]

   b. How much should there be?   [none at all] 1 2 3 4 5 6 7 [maximum]

2. The *opportunity to do important and worthwhile things* in my job:

   a. How much is there now?   [none at all] 1 2 3 4 5 6 7 [maximum]

   b. How much should there be?   [none at all] 1 2 3 4 5 6 7 [maximum]

3. The *self-fulfillment* a person gets from being in my hospital job (that is, being able to use one's own unique capabilities, realizing one's potentialities):

   a. How much is there now?   [none at all] 1 2 3 4 5 6 7 [a very great deal]

   b. How much should there be?   [none at all] 1 2 3 4 5 6 7 [a very great deal]

4. The *opportunity* in my job *to work closely with likeable people*:

   a. How much is there now?   [none at all] 1 2 3 4 5 6 7 [maximum]

   b. How much should there be?   [none at all] 1 2 3 4 5 6 7 [maximum]

5. The *understanding of others on my unit* of the problems and difficulties faced in my job:

   a. How much is there now?   [none at all] 1 2 3 4 5 6 7 [maximum]

   b. How much should there be?   [none at all] 1 2 3 4 5 6 7 [maximum]

6. The *opportunity* in my hospital job *to give help to other people*:

   a. How much is there now?   [none at all] 1 2 3 4 5 6 7 [maximum]

   b. How much should there be?   [none at all] 1 2 3 4 5 6 7 [maximum]

7. The *authority to direct others* connected with my hospital job:

   a. How much is there now?   [none at all] 1 2 3 4 5 6 7 [maximum]

   b. How much should there be?   [none at all] 1 2 3 4 5 6 7 [maximum]

8. The *opportunity* in my hospital job *to share in the determination of methods and procedures*:

   a. How much is there now?   [none at all] 1 2 3 4 5 6 7 [maximum]

   b. How much should there be?   [none at all] 1 2 3 4 5 6 7 [maximum]

9. The *opportunity* in my hospital job *to share in the setting of goals*:

   a. How much is there now?   [none at all] 1 2 3 4 5 6 7 [maximum]

   b. How much should there be?   [none at all] 1 2 3 4 5 6 7 [maximum]

10. Taking everything together, the amount of satisfaction I get from my job:

    a. How much is there now?   [none at all] 1 2 3 4 5 6 7 [maximum]

    b. How much should there be?   [none at all] 1 2 3 4 5 6 7 [maximum]

G. COLLECTION OF COST DATA

Directions to data collectors:

The data collected in this questionnaire will provide information regarding the cost of care on this unit and are for later use in evaluation. The data should be collected by the NAP team member with the person who best knows your hospital accounting and payroll systems. A specific format for collecting the data is not provided as hospitals vary in accounting procedures, but specific cost items are suggested.

IV G
Collection of Cost Data

When considering a change in nursing assignment patterns, an important consideration will be the difference in cost. To make an accurate comparison you will need a record of unit costs prior to a change and a means of obtaining the same unit cost data after the change. If you have an already well-established system of determining operating costs for the patient unit under study, no further data need be collected. If your system provides costs for services but not for patient units within those services, you will have to develop your own format for recording data based on what is available to you. It is important to make this determination NOW so that you will have the data necessary to make later comparisons. The notes below will give you some guidance if you need to organize your own data base.

What costs to include. Patient unit costs are made up of direct and indirect costs. Direct costs are those which buy resources used directly on the unit (mainly unit staff and unit supplies); indirect costs are a fair portion of the costs which buy resources used by several units (nursing office staff, float pool, maintenance, controller's office, etc.). Ideally your cost measure will include all costs which may vary as a result of a change in assignment pattern. This would usually include all direct labor costs and those indirect costs which might go up or down with a change in assignment pattern. Including costs which won't change with a change in assignment pattern doesn't cause much of a problem, since adding a constant to both the "before" costs and the "after" costs won't change the result. Nevertheless, it's good to keep them separate if you can, because something else (e.g., a decision to subcontract housekeeping services) may cause an increase or decrease in these costs.

Costs vary in how much they might change with a change in NAP. Some costs are almost certain to be affected by a different NAP. Changing to an all-RN staff is bound to increase RN costs and decrease LPN costs. Other costs quite likely will change. If increased staffing decreases the demand on the float pool, staff costs increase and float pool costs decrease. Another set of costs may possibly change. Increased nurse accountability may possibly decrease supply costs. When you are designing your cost measure, be sure you include the

"almost certain to be affected" costs, and try to include the "quite likely will be affected" costs. The "may possibly be affected" costs are less important and no special effort should be made to include them.

Costs of what. A moment's thought will help clarify this important issue. Do you want to know cost per day or week or month of operating the unit? Nursing cost per patient day? Nursing cost per admission? Reducing length of stay will reduce cost per admission, but may increase cost per patient day. When census is increasing, unit operating costs might be going up when cost per patient day is declining. It makes sense to gather data that will let you calculate all three costs: unit operating costs, costs per patient day, and costs per admission. Use your hospital's shortest accounting period (one week, two weeks, one month, 1/13 of a year) as the basis for recording unit operating costs, and gather census and admission data that will let you calculate the other two.

How to gather the data. Make your needs clear to someone who knows your hospital accounting and payroll systems. Decide if you will include all, part, or no fringe costs in defining your payroll costs. Decide if you will add up actual costs (how much Stella Jones, Birdie Simmons, Prunella Flook, and so on, are paid) or whether you will add up hours or full-time equivalents (FTEs) and estimate costs (how many RN hours at $7.93/hr., etc.). Decide which indirect costs you will include. A good rule here is exclude them when your portion remains the same regardless of your use. Decide how you will accumulate census and admission data that will let you calculate unit cost per patient day and unit cost per admission.

Working with the accounting and payroll person, set up a data gathering system that will let you accumulate the cost data necessary, and gather them for approximately a 3-month period.

Be absolutely certain that all your key decisions discussed above are in writing, so that exactly comparable data can be gathered in the future.

V

CODING INSTRUCTIONS

This section includes the instructions for counting, digesting and displaying the data collected. Coding is time-consuming and it may be viewed as a clerical chore. Don't view it that way. Coding is an excellent opportunity to find "strange" data and to seek corrections, if needed, or interpretations before it is displayed. You will be wise to have members of the NAP team share the coding responsibility.

Note that the display sheets and worksheets accompanying the coding instructions will need to be copied, as they are used repeatedly. One set, at least, will be needed per unit. These display and worksheets will be the backbone of your analysis.

As previously noted, you will have more reliable data if the Staff Nurse Questionnaire is coded outside the hospital. The coding instructions for that questionnaire (Section V F) should be provided to whoever does the coding.

A. Nursing Assignment Questionnaire
Coding Instructions

For *each* unit, you will abstract data off the questionnaires according to the instructions below. When you are done, you will have per unit:

1 NCI, CMI & PDI Worksheet (Figure V A:1)
1 Nursing Assignment Display Sheet (Figure V A:2)
1 Histogram of NCI(v) (Figure V A:3)
1 NCC Worksheet (Figure V A:4)
4 Questionnaire pages (pp. 3, 4, 5, and 6) of summary data
1 "Group" Coordination Practices Chart

A. Nursing Care Integration (NCI)

Source: Q 1-18, *all* questionnaires for each unit.

1. For *each* of 15* patients, and recording on the NCI, CMI & PDI Worksheet (Figure V A:1):

   a) Count the number of different initials plus "s" and "o"** in each patient's column. This number should be put in Column a of the Worksheet. Do this for each patient, renumbering the questionnaire columns as needed to match the Worksheet patient numbers.

   b) Count the number of boxes in which the most common initial appears. This number goes in Column b. (Also write this initial below the appropriate column on p. 3 of the questionnaire.)

   c) Count the total boxes for each patient that contain the initials "s" or "o". This number goes in Column c.

   d) Calculate Nursing Care Integration *for each patient* (NCI'), by dividing c into b. In algebraic terms, NCI' = b/c.

---

*Or whatever the total is.
**In this step, count *all* "o's", however noted (o, therapist, dietician, etc.) as *one* care-giver. Do not count them individually.

2. Average all NCI' scores. This average is NCI. Record it on the Nursing Assignment Display Sheet (Figure V A:2) on the Nursing Care Integration Scale.

   This care integration index describes how much care is given by a single person (Maximum value = 1).

3. Display the range of variation in Column a for all patients on the NCI(v) histogram (Figure V A:3). See example, below:

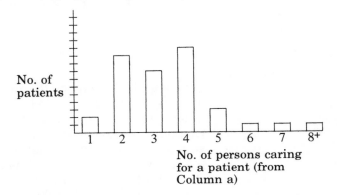

No. of patients

No. of persons caring for a patient (from Column a)

This example of a histogram (or bar chart) shows variation in NCI on a patient unit. The height of each bar indicates the number of patients receiving care from that number of care-givers.

B. Care Management Integration (CMI)

Source: Q 23, *all* questionnaires for each unit.

1. For *each* patient, and recording on the NCI, CMI & PDI Worksheet:

   Count the number of different initials (include "s" and "o") appearing for each patient in this question. This number goes in Column d.

2. Obtain an average for all the numbers in Column d. This is the degree of Care Management Integration (CMI). Record this on the Nursing Assignment Display Sheet.

This is the Care Management Integration index and is based on a count of the number of people sharing in the care management process (Maximum value = 5).

3. Use a copy of questionnaire page 5 as a worksheet and record from the questionnaires the comments under Q 23. Keep this with the other worksheets.

C. Plan-Do Integration (PDI)

Source: Q 23 and Q 1–18.

1. For each of the patients, and recording on the NCI, CMI & PDI Worksheet:

Calculate the value of Plan-Do Integration per patient (PDI') in the following manner:

a) Compare the initials appearing in Q 1–18 with those appearing in Q 23.

b) Count the initials in Q 1–18 that are *not* in Q 23. Do not cound "o". This number goes in Column e.

c) Subtract e from a, then divide that result by a. In algebraic terms, PDI' = (a – e)/a.

2. Obtain an average for all patients of PDI'. This is Plan-Do Integration (PDI). Record this on the Nursing Assignment Display Sheet.

This measure of the integration of planning and doing care counts the number of doers who are not planning, but not viceversa. Using only this score (doers not planning) simplifies the calculation, and, more important, avoids a low degree of PDI in cases where personnel from other shifts are involved in the care management process (Maximum value = 1).

D. Nursing Care Continuity (NCC)

Source: Q 20–21, "CONTINUITY," (last column, Q 1–18); all questionnaires for each unit.

1. For all questionnaires:

a) Record on the NCC Worksheet (Fig. V A:4) how many times "1," "2," "3," etc., appear in the continuity column. When a range is given, use the midpoint of the range if the midpoint is a whole number, e.g., use 5 if the range is 4–6. Use the first whole number *below* the midpoint if the midpoint is not a whole number, e.g., use 4 if the range is 4–5, or 3–6.

b) Total for all questionnaires how many times each number appears, and record in Column b.

c) Multiply the number (Column a) by the times it appears (Column b), and record in Column c. For example, if "4" appears 12 times in the continuity column of all questionnaires, then 4 x 12 = 48, and "48" should be put in Column c, row 4, of the worksheet.

d) Total separately Column b and Column c. Divide the Column c total by the Column b total. This is Nursing Care Continuity (NCC).

e) Record NCC on the Display Sheet on the "Nursing Care Continuity" scale. This care continuity index shows the average care-giver continuity over a seven-day period.

2. Find the most common number, the one with the highest number of entries in Column b, and divide the number of times it appears (the Column b entry) by the total for Column b. This, multiplied by 100, is the percent of patients to which this most common number of care-givers applies. Record the percent figure on the Display Sheet above the most common number.

3. Use a copy of questionnaire page 4 as a worksheet and add from the other questionnaires the checks and circles on Q 22. Keep this with the other worksheets.

E. Care Management Continuity (CMC)

Source: Q 24, all questionnaires for each unit.

1. For all questionnaires:

   a) Calculate an average response for all patients per unit, counting T as "1."

   b) Calculate an average of the three averages. This is Care Management Continuity (CMC). This index records the average number of persons or groups managing a patient's care over a seven-day period.

2. Count the number of T's, and divide by the total number of patients. This result, multiplied by 100, is the percent of patients whose care is managed by a single person or care team for their total stay on the unit; it will be referred to as CMC%.

3. Record CMC on the Display Sheet in the Care Management Continuity scale. Record CMC% above the "1" at the right end of the scale.

F. Care Management Continuity across settings (CMCt)

Source: Q 25, all questionnaires.

1. Use a copy of p. 6 from the questionnaire as your worksheet.

   a) Count the total Yes responses for the three questions on all questionnaires.

   b) Count the total Yes *and* No responses on all questionnaires.

   c) Divide the number of Yes responses by the *total* number of responses, and multiply the result by 100. This measure is Care Management Continuity across settings (CMCt); it indicates the continuing responsibility of unit personnel for patients transferred to or from the unit.

   d) Record CMCt on the Display Sheet in the Care Management Continuity [t] scale.

G. Instructions for Coordination Variables

Source: Q 26 and NCI, CMI & PDI Worksheet.

The purpose of collecting data on coordination in the Nursing Assignment Questionnaire is twofold:
— to let you begin an analysis of the coordination elements of your nursing assignment pattern.
— to let you clarify current coordination practices.

1. Concensus on Current Coordination Practices

   a) Have the people who filled out Q 26 meet together to reach consensus and identify possible problem areas, by creating a group-level Coordination Practices Chart. This group chart will be based on a discussion of your individual responses. Use a blank copy of Q 26 to note the consensus, marking it "GROUP."

   b) Stay focused on describing what *is*, not what should be or what is supposed to be, until consensus is reached. If there is considerable disagreement, determine first if it is semantic (different meanings attached to the same phrases), and sort those out. If disagreement remains, it is substantive and shows honest differences in perception. These are worth noting on the group chart. When key people disagree on how coordination is currently being achieved, problems can arise in organizations. Develop specific statements of the disagreement, agree on data that could resolve it, and how it should be gathered.

   Look for inconsistencies in the data. For example, P-1 or P-2 (Physician as focal person) rarely belongs in Box e (Nursing Coordination); similarly, M-1 (directly doing activities) really makes sense only in Box i (Nursing Coordination).

   c) After filling out the group chart, determine if the relative emphasis shown in the "Degree of Activity" column fits with the importance which *should* be attached to these areas of coordination.

d) Look at the four aspects of coordination, again letting your thinking focus on "what should be," not on "what is." (See Sections VI G, H, and I for some "should be" indicators.)

e) Make notes of your key observations and ideas for change; consider whether having others go through this same analysis process will facilitate making changes in coordination elements of the nursing assignment patterns.

2. Specifying Current Coordination Elements of the Nursing Assignment Pattern

Using the group chart from step b above, code current coordination elements.

a) Nursing Coordination (NC)

1) Box i contains the important response for coding NC.

Using the following codes, record the type of Nursing Coordination in Box j of the group chart as appropriate. In addition, check the appropriate Nursing Care Coordination box on the Nursing Assignment Display Sheet.

M-1 = autonomy
M-2 = consultation
M-4 = hierarchy
M-3 = suggests a constrained level of autonomy

2) Box e indicates whether Nursing Coordination is primarily achieved at:

P-3 = individual level
P-4 = team level
P-5 = unit level

Record individual level, team level or unit level in Box e of the group chart, as appropriate.

b) Care-Cure and Patient Services Coordination

1) Care-Cure Coordination(CCC)

Boxes f and j are the important responses for coding CCC.

Box f:
P-1 & P-2 = key physician role
P-3 = key individual role
P-4 = key team level role
P-5 = key unit level role
Box j:
M-1 = not relevant
M-2 & M-4 = proactive role
M-3 = reactive role
Proactive coordination is P-3, P-4 or P-5 with M-2 or M-4. Specifically nurse proactive coordination would be P-3 or P-4. Reactive (or "passive") coordination is P-1 or P-2 with M-2, M-4, or M-3. Record proactive or reactive in Box j of the group chart as appropriate. Record nurse (P-3 or P-4) or unit level (P-5) in Box f as appropriate. In addition, check the appropriate Care-Cure Coordination box on the Display Sheet.

2) Patient Services Coordination(PSC)

Boxes g and k are the important responses for coding PSC.

Box g:
P-1 & P-2 = key physician role
P-3 = key individual role
P-4 = key team level role
P-5 = key unit level role
P-6 = decide whether this is unit level (e.g., ward clerk, unit manager) or external to unit
Box k:
M-1 = not relevant
M-2 & M-4 = proactive role
M-3 = reactive role
Proactive coordination is P-3, P-4 or P-5 with M-2 or M-4. Specifically nurse proactive coordination would be P-3 or P-4. Reactive coordination is all other combinations of codes.

Record proactive or reactive in Box k as appropriate. Record nurse or unit level in Box g as appropriate. In addition, check the appropriate box for Patient Services Coordination on the Display Sheet.

3) Note: All other responses not shown above should be reviewed to determine the type of nursing coordination, whether proactive or reactive (see definition, footnote to Figure I:1).

c) Inter-shift Coordination (ISC)

1) Box p is the important response for coding ISC.

V-1	= integrated records
V-2	= special care plans
V-3	= oral reports
V-6	= standard care plans

V-4 & V-5	= should be reviewed to determine whether the vehicle for inter-shift coordination is closest to V-1, V-2, V-3 or V-6.

2) Record integrated record, special care plan, oral report or standard care plan in Box p as appropriate. Note: Coding of ISC may be difficult, due to the reporting of several vehicles for conveying information. Use this rule of thumb for making choices between them: "Which one of them is really depended on most heavily?"

Attach the group chart to the Nursing Assignment Display Sheet. In discussions of the assignment pattern, this supporting page is a useful source of data.

Figure V A:1
NCI, CMI & PDI Worksheet

Unit _____

Patient		b	c	b/c		d		a	e	[(a–e)/a]		
1												
2												
3												
4												
5												
6												
7												
8												
9												
10												
11												
12												
13												
14												
15												
Total												
Average												

NCI   CMI   PDI

Figure V A:2
Nursing Assignment Display Sheet

Unit _____

INTEGRATION

Nursing Care Integration   ← lo   hi →

.25   .3   .4   .5   .6   .7   .8   .9   1.0

Care Management Integration   ← lo   hi →

5   4   3   2   1

Plan-Do Integration   ← lo   hi →

.1   .2   .3   .4   .5   .6   .7   .8   .9   1.0

CONTINUITY

Nursing Care Continuity   ← lo   hi →

6   5   4   3   2   1

Care Management Continuity   ← lo   hi →

6   5   4   3   2   1

Care Management Continuity [t] ← lo   hi →

0   25   50   75   100

COORDINATION

Nursing Coordination

☐ hierarchy   ☐ consultation   ☐ autonomy

Care-Cure Coordination

☐ by unit   (passive)   ☐ by nurse   ☐ by unit   (active)   ☐ by nurse

Patient Services Coordination

☐ by unit   (passive)   ☐ by nurse   ☐ by unit   (active)   ☐ by nurse

Inter-Shift Coordination

☐ oral report   ☐ standard care plans   ☐ special care plans   ☐ integrated record

Figure V A:3
Histogram of NCI (v)

Unit _____

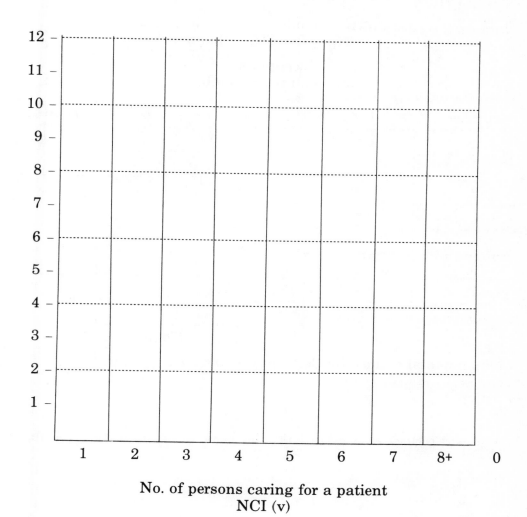

No. of
patients

No. of persons caring for a patient
NCI (v)

Figure V A:4
NCC Worksheet

Unit _____

How often a number appears in Q 20–21,
CONTINUITY Column

a Number	Questionnaire Administration Number:* 1	2	3	b Total	c Column a times Column b
1					
2					
3					
4					
5					
6					
7					
8					
			Total		

Column c total divided by Column b total = NCC

*Draw in extra columns as necessary if the questionnaires are administered more than three times.

B. Patient Characteristics Questionnaire Coding Instructions

This section is written primarily for simple data tabulation, manipulation, and display; therefore several item scores are aggregated to facilitate ease in displaying data on a unit-by-unit level. More complex manipulation by computer is possible and may be desirable when many cross-unit comparisons are made. However, for the use of the questionnaire envisaged in this manual, hand tabulation is simpler and preferable.

For *each* unit, you will abstract data off the Patient Characteristics Questionnaire according to the following instructions. When you are done you will have per unit:

1 - page 1 of these coding instructions
1 - Patient Characteristics Display Sheet (Figure V B:1)
1 - Instability Worksheet (Figure V B:2)
1 - Variability of Process Worksheet (Figure V B:3)
1 - Variability of Therapy Worksheet (Figure V B:4)
1 - Patient Characteristics Questionnaire Worksheet (Figure IV B:1, originally attached to the questionnaire itself)

Source: All questionnaires for a unit.

A. Age

Count and record below the number of patients in each age category.
Infant: 0–1 years _____
Child: 2–12 years _____
Adolescent: 13–20 years _____
Adult: 21–65 years _____
Elderly: 66+ years _____

Chart a histogram of the age distribution on the Patient Characteristics Display Sheet (Figure V B:1).

B. Sex

Chart a histogram of the number of males and females on the Patient Characteristics Display Sheet.

C. Length of stay on unit

Total on the questionnaire the number of days on the unit (actual + expected) per patient, using the following categories:
Less than 24 hours = 0 days
$\geqslant$ 24 but < 48 hours = 1 day
$\geqslant$ 48 but < 72 hours = 2 days
Etc., up to $\geqslant$ 99 days = 99 days

Calculate the average total duration of stay on the unit for the sample of patients. Record the average (mean) and the range on the Patient Characteristics Display Sheet.

D. Instability

1. *Degree of predictable change in condition*

Assign the following weights to the responses:
Less than once per day = 1
Twice per day = 2
Once per shift = 3
A few times per shift = 4
Every hour or more = 5

Record the weight for each patient on the Instability Worksheet (Figure V B:2). Do the same for the following questions.

2 & 3. *Progressive change in condition*

Assign the following weights to the responses:

2. Yes = not weighted
   No = not weighted

3.   good = –1
                       fair = 0
                     poor = 1
                serious = 2
                critical = 3
                 dying = 4
   never transferred = 5

4. *Frequency of emergencies*

Assign the following weights to the responses:
Less than once a week = 1
About once a week = 2
Once every day or two = 3
About once every shift = 4
At least a few times per shift = 5

E. 1. Variability of Process Requirements

Total the check marks *across each row* for all questionnaires and record on the Variability of Process Worksheet (Figure V B:3). Do this for each subcategory of process requirements (basic care conditions, psychological needs, etc.). DO NOT COUNT "DON'T KNOW" (DK). Assign the following weights to the total number of patients in each row and record on Figure V B:3.

No. of patients	Weight
0 or DK	0
1	1
2	2
3	3
4	4
5	5
6	6
7	7
8	8
9	7
10	6
11	5
12	4
13	3
14	2
15	1

Note: These weights assume a sample size (N) of *15* patients. If your sample does not equal 15, weights should be adjusted so that the weights increase up to the *median** of the sample size and then decrease to 1 or 0. Write in new weights as necessary. This weighting system gives the highest possible score to units whose patients are least uniform (half are unlike the other half) and gives the lowest possible score to units whose patients are all alike in their requirements. The highest weight should equal or approximate the median of the sample size.

Calculate the mean (average) weight for each subcategory in the following manner:

Total the row weights. This is w.

Subtract the number of empty and "DK" rows (weight = 0) from the total number of rows (n). This is y. (This is done to eliminate categories which are not represented in the sample; variability is thus measured only in relevant categories of care requirements.)

Divide w by y to get the mean weight for each subcategory. (The possible range for this mean is between 0 and 8, when N = 15.)

Calculate the mean weight for the total sample:

Total all the w's from the subcategories. This total is W.

Total all the y's from the subcategories. This total is Y.

Divide W by Y to obtain the mean sample weight.

To obtain a standardized unit score, divide the mean sample weight by the *median* of the sample (the highest weight possible).

Record this standardized score of the Variability of Process Requirements on the Patient Characteristics Display Sheet

E. 2. Variability of Therapy Requirements

Follow the directions for coding E.1., Variability of Process Requirements. Use the Variability of Therapy Worksheet (Figure V B:4) for recording and calculating. Record the standardized score for Variability of Therapy Requirements on the Patient Characteristics Display Sheet.

It is recommended that the two variability indices not be combined into a single score because studies have shown them to differ significantly on the same units. Retain the worksheets to identify sources of variability within subcategories of the process and therapy requirements. In using the results, variability in either of the two indices may be applied in the selection of propositions, depending on which variable score is highest.

F. Uncertainty

a. Predictability

1. Process requirements

Calculate the percent of all a patient's needs which are predictable by counting the total number of needs of a patient, dividing that by the number of predictable (or circled) needs, and multiplying by 100. Record this percent of predictable needs for each patient on the questionnaires, p. 8, Question F.a)1. Then calculate the mean (average) percent for the total sample of patients.

2. Therapy requirements

Calculate the percent of predictable (circled) therapies (Question F.a)2.) for each patient as described above for process requirements, and calculate the mean percent for the total sample.

Total the percentages for process and therapy and divide by two to obtain the Predictability score. Record on Patient Characteristics Display Sheet.

---

*The median is the number closest to the middle of the range; for example, the median of 15 is 7.5 (which is rounded up to 8), of 20 is 10.

b. *Complexity of processing*

1. Assign the following weights to the responses to Question 1.

very high importance =	100
high =	75
moderate =	50
fair =	25
little or no importance =	0

Calculate the mean weight or score for the total sample of patients.

2–4. Calculate the mean scores for the total sample of patients for Questions 2–4.

5–6. Assign the following weights to Questions 5 & 6.

No. of Problems	Weight
0	0
1	20
2	40
3	60
4	80
5 or more	100

Calculate the mean score for the total sample of patients.

Sum the mean scores for Questions 1–6 and divide this sum by 6 to obtain an index of the Complexity of Processing which will range between 0 and 100. Record on Patient Characteristics Display Sheet.

c. *Complex task integration*

Source: Patient Characteristics Questionnaire Worksheet, attached to the questionnaire (Figure IV B:1).

Using the spaces marked "Complex process integration," check the columns of those patients having (one or more) needs in *at least four* process requirements subcategories.

Using the spaces marked "Complex therapy integration," check the columns of those patients having (one or more) needs in *at least four* therapy requirements subcategories.

In the spaces marked "Complex process and therapy integration," check the columns of those patients who meet *both* of the above criteria.

Record the total number of patients who meet *both* criteria in the space marked "Complex Task Integration." Sum these totals for all patients to obtain the total number of patients requiring complex task integration. Standardize this total by dividing it by the total sample size (N). This is the unit score for Complex Task Integration and it will range from 0 to 1. Record it on the Patient Characteristics Display Sheet.

G. Standardization

Assign the following weights to the responses:

yes, for all aspects =	10
yes, for most aspects =	8
yes, for many aspects =	6
yes, for some aspects =	4
yes, for a few aspects =	2
no, nothing standardized =	0

Calculate the mean (average) score for the sample of patients. This will range between 0 and 10. Record this score on the Patient Characteristics Display Sheet.

H. Multiple Learning Needs

Source: Patient Characteristics Questionnaire Worksheet

Record the number of patients who have *at least* 3 learning needs. Record in space marked "Multiple Learning Needs."

Sum these numbers from all questionnaires, and divide by the total patient sample (N). Record on the Patient Characteristics Display Sheet (Range 0–1).

I. Multiple Technical Requirements

Source: Patient Characteristics Questionnaire Worksheet

Record in the space marked, "Multiple Technical Requirements," the number of patients in each questionnaire who:
1) require at least five (5) technical therapies, *and* who *also*
2) require either
    a total of four or more mechanical therapies,
  or
    any one of the following specific mechanical therapies:
      monitor/respirator
      hemodialysis
      peritoneal dialysis
      stryker frame (with or without traction)
      new tracheostomy

Sum these numbers from all questionnaires, and divide by the total patient sample (N). Record on the Patient Characteristic Display Sheet (Range 0–1).

J. Multiple Coordination Needs

   Source: Patient Characteristics Questionnaire Worksheet

   Record the number of patients who require at least (4) patient care services. Record in space marked "Multiple Coordination Needs."

   Sum these numbers from all questionnaires, and divide by the total patient sample (N). Record on the Patient Characteristic Display Sheet (Range 0–1).

Check that the unit's score on each variable is on the Patient Characteristics Display Sheet. Attach all worksheets to the Display Sheet.

Figure V B:1
Patient Characteristics Display Sheet

Unit _____

A. Age

				-15	Number
				-10	of
				-5	Patients

Infant	Child	Adolescent	Adult	Elderly
0–1 yrs.	2–12 yrs.	13–20 yrs.	21–65 yrs.	66+ yrs.

B. Sex

-15 Number
-10 of
-5   Patients

male   female

C. Mean length of
   stay on unit

← lo   hi →

1 2 3 4 5 6 7 8 9 10 11 12 13 14 15+   days

Range: _____ to _____ days

D. Instability

← lo   hi →

1 2 3 4 5 6 7 8 9 10 11 12 13 14 15
                                                points

E. Variability

Process
Requirements

← lo   hi →

0   .1   .2   .3   .4   .5   .6   .7   .8   .9   1.0
                                              points

Therapy
Requirements

0   .1   .2   .3   .4   .5   .6   .7   .8   .9   1.0
                                              points

F. Uncertainty Factors

   Predictability

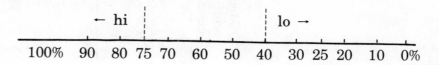

   Complexity of
   Processing

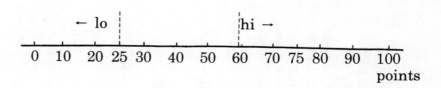

   Complex Task
   Integration

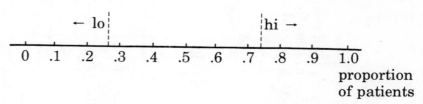

G. Standardization

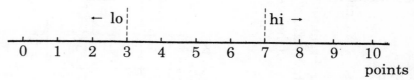

H. Multiple
    Learning
    Needs

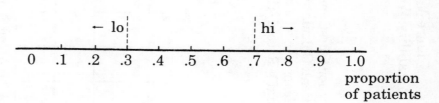

I. Multiple
    Technical
    Requirements

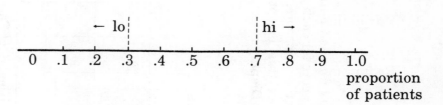

J. Multiple
    Coordination
    Needs

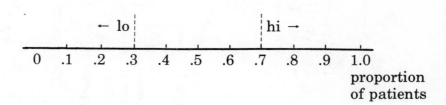

Figure V B:2
Instability Worksheet

Unit ―――――――

Total the weights for each patient for Questions 1–4 renumbering the patients as needed. This total is the score for each patient. Calculate the average (mean) score for the sample of patients. This is the unit score. (Mean scores for *each* of the questions may also be calculated for the unit, but this is optional.) Record the unit Instability score on the Patient Characteristics Display Sheet.

	1	2	3	4	5	6	7	8	9	10	11	12	13	14	15			Mean score per question
									Patients									
1. Predictable change																—	—	
2 & 3. Progressive change in condition																		
4. Frequency of emergencies																		
Total patient scores																		

Total of all Patient Scores ÷ Total Number of Patients (N) = Unit Score

Figure V B:3
Variability of Process Worksheet

Unit _____

Categories	Row #	Total Number of Patients per Row	Weights	Total Row Weights	y (n-# empty & DK rows)	Mean Weight (w/y)	Standard-ized Score
Basic care conditions	1				(n=10)		
	2						
	3						
	4						
	5						
	6						
	7						
	8						
	9						
	10			(w)	(y)		
Psychological needs	1				(n=7)		
	2						
	3						
	4						
	5						
	6						
	7			(w)	(y)		
Social needs	1				(n=5)		
	2						
	3						
	4						
	5			(w)	(y)		
Learning needs	1				(n=7)		
	2						
	3						
	4						
	5						
	6						
	7			(w)	(y)		
Spiritual needs	1				(n=1)		

Note: n = number of rows in each category
N = sample size

Total (W) Total (Y) Mean Sample Weight (W/Y)
[N =   ]

Figure V B:4
Variability of Therapy Worksheet

Unit _____

Categories	Row #	Total Number of Patients per Row	Weights	Total Row Weights	y (n–# empty & DK rows)	Mean Weight (w/y)	Standard-ized Score
Basic care therapies	1				(n=5)		
	2						
	3						
	4						
	5			(w)	(y)		
Technical therapies	1				(n=12)		
	2						
	3						
	4						
	5						
	6						
	7						
	8						
	9						
	10						
	11						
	12			(w)	(y)		
Mechanical therapies	1				(n=9)		
	2						
	3						
	4						
	5						
	6						
	7						
	8						
	9			(w)	(y)		
Observational requirements	1				(n=4)		
	2						
	3						
	4			(w)	(y)		

(n=16)

Categories	Row #	Total Number of Patients per Row	Weights	Total Row Weights	y (n–# empty & DK rows)	Mean Weight (w/y)	Standard-ized Score
Patient care services	1				(n=16)		
	2						
	3						
	4						
	5						
	6						
	7						
	8						
	9						
	10						
	11						
	12						
	13						
	14						
	15						
	16			(w)	(y)		

Note: n = number of rows in each category   Total   Total   Mean Sample Weight
         N = sample size   (W)   (Y)   (W/Y)
                                                                                                      [N =   ]

C. Nursing Resources Questionnaire Coding Instructions

Staffing Record

From the Staffing Record table on p. 2 of the Nursing Resources Questionnaire, calculate the following indices per unit: (1) mix by shift ratio, (2) RN/staff ratio by shift, (3) RN/patient ratio by shift, and (4) average daily absenteeism rate for RNs, LPNs, Aides. The use of a hand calculator is recommended.

Example:

AVERAGE NUMBER OF NURSING PERSONNEL PER SHIFT BY LEVELS AND AVERAGE PATIENT CENSUS FOR WEEKS 1–5

	Week #1	Week #2	Week #3	Week #4	Week #5
Average number of RNs/shift:					
Days	5.0	2.2	3.4	3.4	2.8
Evenings	2.0	2.0	2.2	1.8	2.0
Nights	1.0	1.0	1.0	1.0	1.0
Average number of RNs Absent/day:	1.0	0.0	0.0	2.0	0.0
Average number of LPNs/shift:					
Days	2.4	2.2	2.4	1.4	2.2
Evenings	0.8	0.8	1.0	1.0	1.0
Nights	0.8	0.4	0.4	0.8	1.0
Average number of LPNs Absent/day:	0.0	0.0	2.0	1.0	3.0
Average number of Aides/shift:					
Days	1.6	1.0	1.6	1.2	1.8
Evenings	1.2	1.2	1.0	1.0	1.0
Nights	0.8	1.6	1.4	1.2	1.0
Average number of Aides Absent/day:	3.0	0.5	0.0	0.2	0.0
Average Daily Census:	36.0	33.0	35.0	32.0	32.0

To Obtain Mix by Shift Ratio:

Steps	*Calculations for Example Shown*
1) Calculate the average number of RNs on the day shift for the five-week period.	5.0 + 2.2 + 3.4 + 3.4 + 2.8 = 14.7 14.7 ÷ 5 = 3.67
2) Calculate the average number of LPNs on the day shift for the five-week period.	2.4 + 2.2 + 2.4 + 1.4 + 2.2 = 10.6 10.6 ÷ 5 = 2.12
3) Calculate the average number of Aides on the day shift for the five-week period.	1.6 + 1.0 + 1.6 + 1.2 + 1.8 = 7.2 7.2 ÷ 5 = 1.44
4) Place the three values obtained above in a ratio that expresses the average number of RNs, LPNs, and Aides on the day shift for the five-week period.	3.67/ 2.12/ 1.44 RNs LPNs Aides
5) Divide each of the three values in the ratio by the number of RNs shown in the ratio. This standardizes the ratio and gives the final expression of mix by shift for the day shift over the five-week period.	3.67 ÷ 3.67 = 1 2.12 ÷ 3.67 = 0.57 1.44 ÷ 3.67 = 0.39

The mix by shift ratio for the day shift in the example is:

$$1 \ / \ 0.57/ \ 0.39$$
RNs LPNs   Aides

6) Repeat the above five steps to calculate the mix by shift ratio for the evening shift.

The mix by shift ratio for the evening shift in the example is:

$$1 \ \ / \ 0.57/ \ 0.67$$
RNs LPNs   Aides

7) Repeat steps 1–5 to calculate the mix by shift ratio for the night shift.

The mix by shift ratio for the night shift is:

$$1 \ / \ 3.4 \ / \ 1.2$$
RNs LPNs   Aides

Record mix ratios for each shift on the Nursing Resources Display Sheet (Figure V C:1).

To Obtain RN/Staff Ratio by Shift:

Steps	*Calculations for Example Shown*
8) Calculate the RN/staff ratio for the day shift by adding the values for LPNs and Aides obtained in step 5.	0.57 + .39 = 0.96 RN/staff ratio for day shift = 1/0.96
9) Calculate the RN/staff ratio for the evening shift by adding the values for LPNs and Aides obtained in step 6.	0.57 + 0.67 = 1.91 RN/staff ratio for evening staff = 1/1.91

10) Calculate the RN/staff ratio for the night shift by adding the values for LPNs and Aides obtained in step 7.

$$3.4 + 1.2 = 4.6$$

RN/staff ratio for night shift = 1/4.6

Record RN/Staff Ratios for each shift on the Nursing Resources Display Sheet.

To Obtain RN/Patient Ratio by Shift:

Steps	*Calculations for Example Shown*

11) Calculate the average number of patients per day for the five-week period.

$$36 + 33 + 35 + 32 + 32 = 168$$
$$168 \div 5 = 33.6$$
Average Patient Census

12) Obtain the RN/patient ratio for the day shift for the five-week period by stating the average number of RNs on the day shift (step 1) *over* the value obtained in step 11. Then standardize the ratio by dividing *both* values by the average number of RNs on the day shift (the value obtained in step 1.

3.67/33.6 = RN/patient ratio for day shift (nonstandardized)

1/9.15 = RN/patient ratio for day shift (standardized)

13) Obtain the RN/patient ratio for the evening shift for the five-week period by stating the average number of RNs on the evening shift (step 2) *over* the value obtained in step 11. Then standardize the ratio by dividing *both* values by the average number of RNs on the evening shift.

2/33.6 = RN/patient ratio for evening shift (nonstandardized)

1/16.8 = RN/patient ratio for evening shift (standardized)

14) Obtain the RN/patient ratio for the night shift for the five-week period by stating the average number of RNs on the night shift (step 3) *over* the value obtained in step 11. Then standardize the ratio by dividing *both* values by the average number of RNs on the night shift.

1/33.6 = RN/patient ratio for night shift (nonstandardized)

1/33.6 = RN/patient ratio for night shift (standardized)

Record the standardized ratios on the Nursing Resources Display Sheet.

To Obtain the Average Daily Absenteeism Rate for Staff:

Steps		*Calculations for Example Shown*			

15) For the average daily absenteeism rate for RNs, add the average daily number of RNs for all shifts to the average daily number of RNs absent for each week.

Wk 1	Wk 2	Wk 3	Wk 4	Wk 5
5.0	2.2	3.4	3.4	2.8
2.0	2.0	2.2	1.8	2.0
1.0	1.0	1.0	1.0	1.0
1.0	0.0	0.0	2.0	0.0
9.0	5.2	6.6	8.2	5.8

Steps	*Calculations for Example Shown*

16) Divide the average daily number of RNs *absent* for each week by the totals obtained in step 15.

$$1 \div 9 = 0.11 \quad 0 \div 5.2 = 0 \quad 0 \div 6.6 = 0 \quad 2.0 \div 8.2 = 0.24 \quad 0 \div 5.8 = 0$$

17) Add the five answers obtained in step 16 and divide by 5. Convert to percent by multiplying by 100.

$$0.11 + 0 + 0 + 0.24 + 0 = 0.35$$

$$.35 \div 5 = 0.7$$

Average daily absenteeism
rate for RNs (7 percent)

18) For the average daily absenteeism rate for LPNs, add the average daily number of LPNs for all shifts to the daily average number of LPNs absent for each week.

Wk 1	Wk 2	Wk 3	Wk 4	Wk 5
2.4	2.2	2.4	1.4	2.2
0.8	0.8	1.0	1.0	1.0
0.8	0.4	0.4	0.8	1.0
0.0	0.0	2.0	1.0	3.0
4.0	3.4	5.8	4.2	7.2

19) Divide the average daily number of LPNs *absent* for each week by the totals obtained in step 18.

$$1.0 \div 4.0 = 0.25 \quad 0 \div 3.4 = 0 \quad 2.0 \div 5.8 = 0.34 \quad 1.0 \div 4.2 = 0.23 \quad 3.0 \div 7.2 = 0.41$$

20) Add the five answers obtained in step 19 and divide by 5. Convert to percent.

$$0.25 + 0 + 0.34 + 0.23 + 0.41 = 1.23$$

$$1.23 \div 5 = 0.24$$

Average daily absenteeism
rate for LPNs (24 percent)

21) For the average daily absenteeism rate for Aides, add the average daily number of Aides for all shifts to the daily average number of Aides absent in each week.

Wk 1	Wk 2	Wk 3	Wk 4	Wk 5
1.6	1.0	1.6	1.2	1.8
1.2	1.2	1.0	1.0	1.0
0.8	1.6	1.4	1.2	1.0
3.0	0.5	0.0	0.2	0.0
6.6	4.3	4.0	3.6	3.8

22) Divide the average daily number of Aides *absent* for each week by the totals obtained in step 21.

$$3.0 \div 6.6 = 0.45 \quad 0.5 \div 4.3 = 0.11 \quad 0 \div 4.0 = 0 \quad 0.2 \div 3.6 = 0.05 \quad 0 \div 3.8 = 0$$

23) Add the five answers obtained in step 22 and divide by 5. Convert to percent.

$$0.45 + 0.11 + 0 + 0.05 + 0 = 0.61$$

$$0.61 \div 5 = 0.12$$

Average daily absenteeism
rate for Aides (12 percent)

24) Have a cup of coffee or tea and relax!

Record average daily absenteeism rate separately for RNs, LPNs, and Aides on the Nursing Resources Display Sheet.

Summary of how the example data would be organized on the **Nursing Resources Display** Sheet:

	Mix by Shift (RN/LPN/Aide)	RN/Staff Ratio (RN/LPN=Aide)
Day	1/0.57/0.39	1/0.96
Eve	1/0.57/0.67	1/1.91
Night	1/3.4/1.2	1/4.6

	RN/Patient Ratio
Day	1/9.15
Eve	1/16.8
Night	1/33.6

Absenteeism

```
                                    ← lo¦              ¦hi →
                                        ¦      RNs     ¦           Aides
        ─────────────────┬──────────────┬──────────────┬──────────────
                %        3%             6%             9%            12%
                                                          LPN = 24%
```

Staffing Instability

From information on the Rotation/Flotation Record and additional information available from steps 1–3 of the mix by shift calculations which have already been done, you will calculate the following: (1) daily average number of RNs floating and rotating to/from day shift for a five-week period, (2) daily average number of LPNs floating and rotating to/from day shift for a five-week period, (3) daily average number of Aides floating and rotating to/from the day shift for a five-week period, (4) RN staffing instability index, (5) LPN staffing stability index, and (6) Aide staffing instability index.

Example:

AVERAGE ROTATION AND FLOTATION SCORES
FOR FIVE-WEEK PERIOD BY LEVEL OF PERSONNEL

	Wk. #1	Wk. #2	Wk. #6	Wk. #4	Wk. #5
Data for RNs:					
1) Average number of RNs floating onto unit during day shift	1	0	1.2	0	0
2) Average number of RNs floating off unit during day shift	0	0	0	1	1
3) Average number of RNs rotating to/from evening shift to/from day shift	0.4	2	3	1	2
4) Average number of RNs rotating to/from night shift to/from day shift	0	1	2	1	2
Data for LPNs:					
5) Average number of LPNs floating onto unit during day shift	0.3	0	1	0	0
6) Average number of LPNs floating off unit during day shift	0	0	0	0	1
7) Average number of LPNs rotating to/from evening shift to/from day shift	1	1	1	0.6	2
8) Average number of LPNs rotating to/from night shift to/from day shift	0	0.5	0	0	1
Data for Aides:					
9) Average number of Aides floating onto unit during day shift	0	0	0	0	0
10) Average number of Aides floating off unit during day shift	0	0	0.2	0	0
11) Average number of Aides rotating to/from evening shift to/from day shift	1	2	0	0	1
12) Average number of Aides rotating to/from night shift to/from day shift	2	0	1	0	0

To Obtain Staffing Instability Indexes

Steps	*Calculations for Example Shown*

25) Calculate the average number of RNs floating onto unit during day shift for five-week period.

$$1 + 0 + 1.2 + 0 + 0 = 2.2$$
$$2.2 \div 5 = 0.02$$

26) Calculate the average number of RNs floating off unit during day shift for five-week period.

$$0 + 0 + 0 + 1 + 1 = 2$$
$$2 \div 5 = 0.4$$

27) Calculate the average number of RNs rotating to/from evening shift to/from day shift for five-week period.

$$0.4 + 2 + 3 + 1 + 2 = 6.2$$
$$6.2 \div 5 = 1.24$$

28) Calculate the average number of RNs rotating to/from night shift to/from day shift for five-week period.

$$0 + 1 + 2 + 1 + 2 = 6$$
$$6 \div 5 = 1.2$$

29) Sum the responses obtained in steps 25–28. This gives you the average daily number of RNs floating and rotating relative to the day shift for five-week period.

$$0.02 + 0.4 + 1.24 + 1.2 = 2.86$$

30) To obtain the RN staffing instability index, divide the value obtained in step 29 by the daily average number of RNs on the day shift for a five-week period (see step 1).

$$2.86 \div 3.67 = 0.77$$
RN staffing instability index

31) Calculate the average number of LPNs floating onto unit during day shift for five-week period.

$$0.3 + 0 + 1 + 0 + 0 = 1.3$$
$$1.3 \div 5 = 0.26$$

32) Calculate the average number of LPNs floating off unit during day shift for five-week period.

$$0 + 0 + 0 + 0 + 1 = 1$$
$$1 \div 5 = 0.2$$

33) Calculate the average number of LPNs rotating to/from evening shift to/from day shift for five-week period.

$$1 + 1 + 1 + 0.6 + 2 = 5.6$$
$$5.6 \div 5 = 1.12$$

34) Calculate the average number of LPNs rotating to/from night shift to/from day shift for five-week period.

$$0 + 0.5 + 0 + 0 + 1 = 1.5$$
$$1.5 \div 5 = 0.3$$

35) Sum the responses obtained in steps 31–34. This gives you the average daily number of LPNs floating and rotating relative to the day shift for a five-week period.

$$0.26 + 0.2 + 1.12 + 0.3 = 1.88$$

Steps	*Calculations for Example Shown*
36) To obtain the LPN staffing instability index, divide the value obtained in step 35 by the daily average number of LPNs on the day shift for a five-week period (see step 2).	$1.88 \div 2.12 = 0.88$ LPN staffing instability index
37) Calculate the average number of Aides floating onto unit during day shift for five-week period.	$0 + 0 + 0 + 0 + 0 = 0$ $0 \div 5 = 0$
42) To obtain the Aide staffing instability index, divide the value obtained in step 41 by the daily average number of Aides on the day shift for a five-week period (see step 3).	$1.44 \div 1.44 = 1$ Aide staffing instability index

Summary of Staffing Instability example data:

RN staffing instability index	0.77 (record as 77%)
LPN staffing instability index	0.88 (record as 88%)
Aide staffing instability index	1.00 (record as 100%)

Record data on Nursing Resources Display Sheet as a percent. Numbers larger than 1.0, say 1.23, should be recorded as "123%" at the right edge of the "Staffing Instability" scales on the Nursing Resources Display Sheet.

Special Training

From the Special Training table in the questionnaire, you will calculate the average number of hours of special training for each person per category.

1) Treat each percent figure in the table as a decimal number (e.g., 40% = .40)

2) Multiply that decimal number by the number of hours spent training each staff member in that special area.

Record the result, the average number of hours of special training per staff member, in the appropriate boxes on the Nursing Resources Display Sheet.

Example:

	RN		LPN		Aides	
	%		%		%	
		hrs.		hrs.		hrs.
a) Documentation	40%		0%		0%	
		8 hrs.		0 hrs.		0 hrs.
b) Nursing process	25%		0%		0%	
		16 hrs.		0 hrs.		0 hrs.
c) Leadership and interpersonal skills	100%		100%		100%	
		90 hrs.		40 hrs.		50 hrs.
d) Facilitating accountability	0%		0%		0%	
		0 hrs.		0 hrs.		0 hrs.
e) Medications	0%		50%		0%	
		0 hrs.		10 hrs.		0 hrs.

Summary of example data on Display Sheet:

	RN	LPN	Aides
a) Documentation	3.2 hrs.	0 hrs.	0 hrs.
b) Nursing process	4.0 hrs.	0 hrs.	0 hrs.
c) Leadership & interpersonal skills	90 hrs.	40 hrs.	50 hrs.
d) Facilitating accountability	0 hrs.	0 hrs.	0 hrs.
e) Medications	0 hrs.	5 hrs.	0 hrs.

Figure V C:1
NURSING RESOURCES DISPLAY SHEET

Unit _____

	Mix by Shift (RN/LPN/Aide)	RN/Staff Ratio (RN/LPN+Aide)	LO:	LPN and Aide more than double the RN number.
Day	_____/_____/_____	_____/_____		
Eve	_____/_____/_____	_____/_____	HI:	RN more than double the LPN and Aide number.
Night	_____/_____/_____	_____/_____		

	RN/Patient Ratio		
Day	_____/_____	LO:	1/9 or more
Eve	_____/_____	HI:	1/3 or less
Night	_____/_____		

Part-time/Full-time Ratio*   _____/_____   LO: 1/4 or more
                                                      HI: 1/1 or less

Staff Commitment:**

```
                    ← lo ┆           ┆ hi →
        ─────────────────────────────────────────
                           0
```

Stability:
a. Turnover

```
                  ← lo ┆      ┆ hi →
        ───────────────────────────────────────
        0%     25%    50%    75%   100%
```

b. Absenteeism

```
                 ← lo ┆       ┆ hi →
        ───────────────────────────────────────
        0       3%     6%     9%    12%
```

c. Staffing Instability

```
                   ← lo ┆      ┆ hi →
   RN   ───────────────────────────────────────
        0%     25%    50%    75%   100%

   LPN  ───────────────────────────────────────
        0%     25%    50%    75%   100%

   Aide ───────────────────────────────────────
        0%     25%    50%    75%   100%
```

Staff Availability*	Scarce	Available	Ample
RN Specialists (BSN)	|⊢_____|_____⊣	
RN: AD & Dip.	⊢_____|_____⊣		
LPN	⊢_____|_____⊣		
Aides	⊢_____|_____⊣		

Preparation Ratio (MSN, BSN/AD, Dip/ LPN, Aide)	_____/_____/_____	LO: 1 MSN or BSN to 10 or more other staff HI: 1 MSN or BSN to 3 other staff
Experience Ratio (MSN, BSN/AD, Dip/ LPN, Aide)	_____/_____/_____	LO: LPN + Aide experience 2 years or more greater than RNs HI: LPN + Aide experience at least a year less than RNs

Special Training

	Average number of hours of special training per staff member		
	RN	LPN	Aides
a. Documentation in charting			
b. Use of nursing process			
c. Leadership and interpersonal skills			
d. Training intended to facilitate individual accountability			
e. Medications			

In-service Education Resource (record summary comment):**

---

*The data for these indexes will be drawn from Section IV E, Data from Director and Nursing Office, and is coded with that data.

**No data collection instrument provided. See "Directions to data collectors," Nursing Resources Questionnaire, for comments regarding commitment and absenteeism.

D. Organizational Support Questionnaire Coding Instructions

A. Medical Resources

1. Physician presence on the unit:

Total the responses to Question A–1, p. 1 of the questionnaire.

Divide this total by the average daily census for the unit calculated in step 11 of the Nursing Resources Questionnaire Coding Instructions.

Record the result on the Organizational Support Display Sheet (Figure V D:1) under "Physician Presence (hours per week per patient)."

2. Physician-Nurse Communication

Using the key below, count the number of checks in the circled boxes, and record that number on the Organizational Support Display Sheet under Physician-Nurse Communication.

2.1 Rounds with doctors:

Regularly used ☐ ⟶ | Nurse primarily collaborates with MD on care plan. ☐

Irregular or none (Go to ☐ | Doctor primarily informs nurse ☐
Question 2.2) | of care plan.

2.2 Scheduled joint educational sessions:

Regularly used ☐ ⟶ | Usually a discussion between nurses and physicians. ☐

Irregular or none (Go to ☐ | Usually lecture by physician ☐
Question 2.3)

| Usually lecture by nurse ☐

2.3 Meetings on the unit:

Regularly used ☐ ⟶ | Usually collaborative discussion of patient care between nurse and physician. ☐

Irregular or none (Go to ☐ | Usually physician provides ☐
Question 2.4) | information to nurse.

| Usually nurse provides ☐
| information to physician.

2.4 Integrated medical record (all health professionals contribute to same progress notes and/or problem list):
Yes ☐   No ☐

3. Physician-Nurse Collegiality

Collect the responses to Q 3 from the Organizational Support Questionnaire.

Using a copy of that page as a worksheet, calculate an average response for each of the 12 boxes shown (4 boxes per question).

Now sum the averages in the far left boxes *down the page* on your worksheet and average those (i.e., divide by 3).

Do the same for the middle left, middle right, and far right boxes. See the example below.

Record these 4 figures in the appropriate boxes (far left, middle left, etc.) under Physician-Nurse Collegiality on the Organizational Support Display Sheet.

If there are significant variations among the answers by your respondents, you will both improve accuracy and facilitate later implementation if these are discussed and clarified among the respondents. If responses to this question change as a result of this discussion, you should recalculate the averages and change the Display Sheet accordingly.

Example:

3.1 Independent functions:

| 5% | 45% | 45% | 5% = 100% |

Physicians recognize only dependent functions as the true nursing role.

Physicians view dependent functions as the primary nurse role.

Physicians recognize independent functions as occasionally important to patient care.

Physicians view independent nursing functions as the primary nurse role.

3.2 Doctor-nurse coordination:

| 5% | 45% | 45% | 5% = 100% |

Physicians expect nurses to only follow orders.

Physicians expect nurses to follow orders and provide relevant information.

Physicians expect nurses to be junior colleagues in some care management decisions.

Physicians view nurses as the expert member of care team for certain care management activities.

3.3 Stereotyping:

| 5% | 95% | 00% | 0% = 100% |

Physicians view all nursing staff as narrowly trained semi-professionals.

Physicians distinguish only between nurses and aides, and rely on familiarity with staff to distinguish ability of nurses.

Physicians recognize differences within the RN group, but are unclear on distinctions related to professional preparation.

Physicians understand and have different expectations of differently trained RNs.

| Sum = 15% | 185% | 90% | 10% |
| ÷ 3 = | ÷ 3 = | ÷ 3 = | ÷ 3 = |

Average =

| 5% | 62% | 30% | 3% |

B. Support Services

1. Unit Support Services

Assign the following weights to the responses to Question B–1, p. 4, averaging the weights if 2 or more responses appear in one box:

Those responsible	*Weight*
U = unit nursing	1
O = other nursing	2
H = other hospital	4
X = not used	0

Availability of coverage	*Weight*
√ = needed but unavailable	–1
box not checked	0

Responsiveness to nursing	*Weight*
G = good	3
F = fair	0
P = poor	–1

You will calculate a separate unit support score for days and weekends, and for evenings and nights, using the Score Sheet for Support Services (Figure V D:2) and the following instructions.

Days and Weekends: Line up the Score Sheet on the right side of the original questionnaire. Recording on the Score Sheet, total *across the page* the scores in columns I and III and subtract for the checks in the "Day" and "Wknd" columns. See example page; the column on the far right marked "Total Weights; Day/Wknd" shows the totals which would be on the Score Sheet.

Evenings and Nights: Repeat the process, subtracting for checks in the "Eve" and "Nite" columns.

Sum both columns on the Score Sheet.

Divide each total by the total number of services used, that is those marked with U, O, or H.

Record the average score on the Score Sheet and on the Organizational Support Display Sheet under Unit Support Services, using an "x" to mark the day/weekend score, and a "y" to mark the evening/night score.

2. Patient Care Support Services

Repeat the procedure used in Unit Support Services (step 1 above) to calculate and record the average scores for Patient Care Services. Again, use the Score Sheet for Support Services.

Code the role of the nurse specialist as staff development, patient care, or consultation on the Score Sheet and on the Organizational Support Display Sheet. Write "none present," if the unit has no nurse specialists.

Make a note of the services which present problems, for later discussion in the nursing management group.

Example:

	I Responsibility for Providing Service U=Unit nursing (RNs, LPNs, Aides) O=Other nursing dept. personnel H=Other hospital departments X=Not used	II Absense of Coverage Place √ only if services are both unavailable and needed				III Responsiveness to Nursing Needs G=Good F=Fair P=Poor	Score Sheet Columns Total Weights; Day/ Wknd	Total Weights; Eve/ Nite
		Day	Wknd	Eve	Nite			

1. Unit Support Services
  a. Technical:
       Specimen collection
	U,H (2.5)		(-1)√	(-1)√		F-G (1.5)	4.0	2.0

Patient transportation	U,O,H,H(2.7)					F-G (1.5)	4.2	4.2
Messenger service	X							
Ordering and stocking supplies	U,H (2.5)					G (3)	5.5	5.5
Laundry stocking & disposal	H (4)				(-1)√	G (3)	7.0	7.0
Unit housekeeping	H (4)					G (3)	7.0	6.0
Unit maintenance	H (4)				(-1)√	F-G (1.5)	5.5	4.5
b. Clerical: Unit records	U,H (2.5)					G (3)	5.5	4.5
Scheduling patients & appointments	U,H (2.5)					G (3)	5.5	5.5
Phone answering	U (1)	(-1)√		(-1)√		F (0)	0	0
Transcribing MDs orders	U,H(2.5)					G (3)	5.5	5.5
Processing unit admissions	U,H (2.5)					G (3)	5.5	5.5
Processing unit discharges	U,H (2.5)					G (3)	5.5	5.5
Receptionist duties	U (1)			(-1)√	(-1)√	G (3)	3.0	3.0
c. Administrative: Recruitment	U (1)					P (-1)	0	0
Staff scheduling	O (2)					G (3)	5.0	5.0
Arranging daily coverage	U (1)					G (3)	4.0	4.0
Patient classification	U (1)					G (3)	4.0	4.0
New nurse orientation	O (2)					F (0)	2.0	2.0
Staff education	O (2)					G (3)	5.0	5.0
Other unit support of administrative functions							104.2	99.2

Total No. Services: ___19___   Total Score: __83%__ __78%__

Day/Wknd Average Score $\dfrac{83.7}{19} = 4.4$ Eve/Nite Average Score $\dfrac{78.7}{19} = 4.1$

C. Physical Environment

Using the responses to Questions C1 and C2, assign a weight from the tables below for each check on the questionnaire.

1. Proximity of materials

	Patient Room	Near All Rooms	Mobile Carts	Central Location But Far From Some Rooms
Clean Linen	(3)	(2)	(1)	(0)
Central Service Supplies	(3)	(2)	(1)	(0)
Medical Records	(3)	(2)	(1)	(0)
Medications	(3)	(2)	(1)	(0)
Waste Disposal	(3)	(2)	(1)	(0)
Linen Disposal	(3)	(2)	(1)	(0)

2. Communication system

	Yes	No
Telephone in or near patient's room for nurse use	(2)	(0)
Pocket pager	(3)	(0)
Intercom and call light from patient's room to nursing station	(2)	(0)
Nurse call light only	(1)	(0)

Sum all weights from *both* questions (range = 0–26).

Record on the Organizational Support Display Sheet under Physical Environment.

Figure V D:1
ORGANIZATIONAL SUPPORT DISPLAY SHEET

Unit _____

Physician Presence (hours per week per patient)

← lo   hi →

0   5   10   15

Physician-Nurse Communication

← lo   hi →

1   2   3   4   5   6   7

Physician-Nurse Collegiality

← lo   hi →

subordinate   assistant   junior colleague   colleague

Unit Support Services: Day/weekend = x
                       Eve/night   = y

← lo   hi →

1   2   3   4   5   6   7

Patient Support Services: Day/weekend = x
                         Eve/night   = y

← lo   hi →

1   2   3   4   5   6   7

Clinical Nurse Specialist Role _____

Physical Environment

← lo   hi →

0   5   10   15   20   25

Financial Constraint:* _____

*This scale will be coded with Data from Director and Nursing Office.

Figure V D:2
Score Sheet for Support Services

Unit _____

1. Unit Support Services

Total Weights Day/Weekend:	Total Weights Evening/Night:

Line up with right side of response page

2. Patient Care Support Services

Total Weights Day/Weekend:	Total Weights Evening/Night:

Line up with right side of response page

Total Score=

	Day/Weekend	Evening/Night		Day/Weekend	Evening/Night
$\dfrac{\text{Total Score}}{\text{No. services}}$ =	_____	_____		_____	_____
AVERAGE SCORE:	_____	_____		_____	_____

* *

Nurse specialist role   staff   patient   resource   other
(check as many as apply):   development _____   care _____   to staff _____   _____

E. Data from Director and Nursing Office Coding Instructions

A. Nursing Resources

Unit Staff Data

Using the instructions below, you will calculate per unit the Preparation Ratio, Experience Ratio, and Part-time Ratio.

Source: Unit Staff Data table, p. 1. of questionnaire.

1. Preparation Ratio

   From the Nursing Education column:

   a) Add all checks in "MSN, BSN" column, counting part-time persons as a half.

   b) Add all checks in "AD, Dip" column, counting part-time as one-half.

   c) Add all checks in "LPN" and "none" columns; count part-time as one-half.

   d) Write the separate totals as a/b/c, for example 0/4.5/7.0, on the Nursing Resources Display Sheet (Figure V C:1).

2. Experience Ratio

   From the Years of Experience on Unit column:

   a) Average the number of years of experience for those persons with checks in the "MSN, BSN" column; count part-time as one-half.

   b) Average the number of years of experience for those with checks in the "Ad, Dip" column; count part-time as one-half.

   c) Average the number of years of experience for those with checks in the "LPN" or "none" columns; count part-time as one-half.

   d) Write the above averages as a/b/c, for example 0/1.3/4.2, on the Nursing Resources Display Sheet.

3. Part-time/Full-time Ratio

   From the Part and Full-time columns:

   a) Total the checks in the "P" column.

   b) Total the checks in the "F" column.

   c) Write as a/b, for example 7/14, on Nursing Resources Display Sheet.

Staff Availability

Source: Staff Availability table

Record on the Nursing Resource Display Sheet under "Staff Availability," the level of availability of each category, adding together RN:AD and RN:Dip.

Unit Staff Turnover

Source: Unit Staff Turnover table.

Staff turnover is a percent figure based on a fraction, of which the numerator is the number of people joining and leaving a unit, and the denominator is the total number of staff. Turnover is usually expressed as *annual* turnover, the number of people joining and leaving over a 12-month period. The formula below uses *six months* of data, but will give an *annual* rate.

1. For RN turnover:

   a) Use the Unit Staff Turnover table. For RNs only, count the New hires + Transfers to + Transfers from + Terminations. This is the numerator for the RN turnover fraction.

   b) Use the Unit Staff Data table, and count all the RNs employed on the unit.

This is the denominator for the RN turnover fraction.

c) Divide a by b and multiply by 100 for the percent annual turnover of RNs.

d) Record under Turnover on Nursing Resource Display Sheet, marking "RN" above appropriate scale point.

2. For LPN turnover:

a) Repeat step a above, using LPN data from the Unit Staff Turnover table.

b) Repeat step b, counting all LPNs listed in Unit Staff Data table.

c) Repeat step c to get the percent annual turnover of LPNs.

d) Record under Turnover on Nursing Resources Display Sheet, marking "LPN" above appropriate scale point.

3. Aide turnover,

Repeat the same four steps as above but use Aide data from the tables to determine percent annual turnover of Aides.

Note 1:
The above is a short version for calculating turnover, using readily available data. The standard way of calculating these turnover figures would have been to use the following:

numerator: No. in job category joining and leaving unit over 12 month period.

denominator: *Sum* of total in job category at beginning of 12 months and total in job category at end of 12 months.

This fraction, expressed as a percent (multiplied by 100), would be the job category's annual turnover.

Note 2:
To calculate total unit turnover, repeat the four-step calculation for the entire group. Taking an average of the three turnover figures will be accurate *only* if there are the same number of RNs as LPNs as Aides.

In-Service Assessment

Source: In-Service Assessment table

Prepare brief summaries of the internal strength (Qs a–c) of the in-service program, of hospital support (Qs d–f) for the program, and of the quality of the orientation program (Q g).

Record summaries on Nursing Resources Display Sheet.

B. Organizational Support

Financial Constraint

Source: Financial Constraint question

Prepare a brief summary of the financial constraint facing the hospital. Calculate an average separately for item 1 and for item 3. Use the general guidelines below to categorize the hospital's level of financial constraint.

	Severe Constraint	Significant Constraint	Normal Constraint
1. Margin of net revenues over (under) expenses, three-year average	net loss	0–1%	Over 1.0%
2. Revenues from third party payers	60% or less	61–80%	Over 80%
3. Hospital occupancy, three-year average	60% or less	61–75%	Over 75%

Record summary on Organizational Support Display Sheet (Figure V D:1).

F. Staff Nurse Questionnaire Coding Instructions

Note: It is not advisable to code the Staff Nurse Questionnaire in the hospital or by hospital personnel. Questionnaires are rarely answered openly when anonymity is not fully protected.

Job Characteristics

Source: Job Characteristics section of questionnaire (skip Background Information section).

Divide the questionnaires into RNs, LPNs, and Aides. Make *sure* there are *at least four* respondents in each category. *Every* analysis group should have *at least four* respondents to assure both the reliability of the results and to protect the respondents' anonymity. Also, avoid reporting any analysis that allows the scores of less than four respondents to be inferred. E.g., if four RNs and two Aides are the respondents, do not report both RN satisfaction and All Respondent satisfaction.

1. For all RN respondents, calculate and record *b minus a* (b–a) for all ten questions. You can use the right hand margin of the questionnaire to note these. For *each* question, average the b–a score of all RN respondents on the unit.

    Average the b–a scores for Q 1–3. Subtract this average from 5. This indicates the level of Intrinsic Satisfaction.

    Average the b–a scores for Q 4–6. Subtract this average from 5. This indicates the level of Interpersonal Satisfaction.

    Average the b–a scores for Q 7–9. Subtract this average from 5. This indicates the level of Involvement Satisfaction.

    Overall satisfaction is indicated by the average of Q 10, subtracted from 5.

2. Repeat the above process for LPNs.

3. Repeat the above process for Aides.

4. Divide *all* the questionnaires into two categories: respondents who have worked less than a year *AND* respondents who have worked a year or more. If there are at least four respondents in *each* of these two categories, repeat the above process.

5. When you have completed the analysis, *destroy the individual questionnaires*. This is required to protect respondent anonymity.

The instrument from which these questions are drawn is described in the article abstracted below:

Munson, F. C. and Heda, S. S. An instrument for measuring nursing satisfaction. *Nursing Research*. March-April, 1974, 23(2):159–166.

To test the validity of a modified instrument designed to measure job satisfaction, based on one presented by Porter (Porter and Lawler, 1965, 1978), 351 registered nurses in 55 patient units in hospitals completed the 22-item, four-factor (intrinsic, involvement, interpersonal, and extrinsic) questionnaire. When answers were subjected to matched-pair correlations, the instrument was found to have properties ascribed to it and to measure job satisfaction as an organizational variable. (Authors' abstract)

VI

CONNECTIVE PROPOSITIONS

This section provides general guidelines to help you interpret the analysis you have made of your patient characteristics, nursing resources, and organizational support. They "connect" or link these variables with the conceptual elements of nursing assignment patterns that have been presented in this manual. The guidelines have been framed in the form of propositions so they can assist you in making recommendations to maintain current patterns or to select new ones.

The connective propositions should be used like a dictionary, as a reference source. They don't mean much if read as other parts of this manual were. Note that because the interrelations among the variables that affect assignment patterns are immensely complex, we have been able to present only the most significant of these interrelations.

In using the propositions you will note that each set has two parts, "Range Attributes" and "Connective Propositions." "Range Attributes" give you a sense of the probable impact an increase or decrease in the element will have on quality, cost, and satisfaction. "Connective Propositions" are the actual listing of the relations between patient characteristics, nursing resources, and organizational support, on the one hand, and the nursing assignment elements on the other.

The propositions are based on the literature in very large part. Numeric references in the right margin identify the literature that was consulted in forming them. Bibliographic annotations for each reference number appear in Appendix 1. In some cases, the propositions also draw on experiences of the project group. When there are no numeric references, the propositions should be assumed to have this source. Since the literature emphasizes quality rather than cost considerations, we have added Section VI J, to help you make cost implications an explicit part of your decision process.

A special note on the patient characteristic, "standardization." For ease of data collection, coding, and display, we have treated standardization of care as a patient characteristic. Standardization is closely linked to patient characteristics. Specifically when predictability of patients is low, standardization cannot be high; but when predictability of patients is high, standardization can be low *or* high. The point is, it can be changed without changing patient characteristics. Standardization is really a characteristic of the organization, a resource that influences assignment patterns much as the physical environment, or physician-nurse collegiality influences them. There it makes sense to treat standardization of care as an organizational support variable, and we do so throughout this chapter.

A. USING THE CONNECTIVE PROPOSITIONS

In this section we outline a method of blending your professional judgment and the connective propositions to reach a nursing assignment pattern decision. This part will concentrate on the mechanics of the process of linking a unit's NAP with patient characteristics, nursing resources, and organizational support. The suggested propositions are intended to aid you in applying your professional judgment and in allowing unit leadership to do the same. Don't view these propositions as equivalent to the coding manual instructions. They are guides, not specifications.

In fact, they cannot be specifications. Unless your situation is very unusual, all the connective propositions for a unit will not point in the same direction. We have placed an * beside those propositions that, in our judgment, are particularly significant. These asterisks are our "judgment calls," and are added only as a convenience to you.

We have also used another code which may be helpful when the nature of the relation is not obvious:

$ — the proposition is primarily related to cost saving.

Q — the proposition is primarily related to the quality or safety of nursing care.

E — the proposition relates primarily to the ease of introducing the NAP element.

Inevitably, you will have reached some tentative judgments about the kind of assignment pattern you think is "right" for the study unit. Try to hold these in abeyance while you work through the process we outline here. Closed minds can neither see alternatives clearly nor weigh them fairly.

You will want to work through your recommendations one unit at a time, considering each element in turn.

1. Make enough copies of the Recommendations Sheet (Figure VI:1) so you have one copy per element per unit (i.e., 8 elements X no. units studied).

   a) Read the NCI Range Attributes.

   b) Turn to NCI Connective Propositions, and, by using your Patient Characteristics, Nursing Resources, and Organizational Support Display Sheets and the NCI(v) bar graph, identify those propositions that are applicable to your unit. Ignore the rest.

   c) Record the applicable propositions on the Recommendations Worksheet (Figure VI:1). We have provided an example of the worksheet filled in for a hypothetical unit in Figure VI:2.

   d) The worksheet should let you pull the facts together, make tentative judgments based on those facts, and record the judgments together with any reasons that may clarify them.

   Note that the example worksheet actually draws on four different sources:

   i. The element's range attributes
   ii. The connective propositions
   iii. Cost chart in Section VI J
   iv. Nurses' professional judgment

Figure VI:1
Recommendations Worksheet

Unit _____

NAP element _____

Relevant Propositions:

Support
for hi _____ (or lo less beneficial)

Support
for lo _____ (or hi less beneficial)

Probable impact on:

	Unit Cost	Cost/ day	Cost/ stay	Quality	Satisfaction RN	other
hi _____						
lo _____						

Notes:

Recommendation:

Figure VI:2
Example of Recommendations Worksheet

Unit ___2N___

NAP element ___NCI___

Relevant Propositions:

Support for hi ___NCI___ (or lo less beneficial)

hi: lo variability

hi: hi patient support services   (Variability = .2)

(Patient support = 5.0)

Support for lo ___NCI___ (or hi less beneficial)

hi less beneficial: hi multiple technical requirements   (Multiple technical requirements = 7.8)

hi less beneficial: geriatric   (11/15, or 73% of patients over 65)

lower: hi instability with lo RN/staff ratio and lo unit support services   (Instability = 11, RN/staff ratio = 1/1.9, Unit Support = 2.3)

lo: hi RN turnover, lo LPN turnover, aides about medium   (Turnover: RN = 76%, LPN = 19%, Aide = 33%)

lo: special training for LPNs   (LPNs: 42 hours training in special care needs of geriatric patients)

Probable impact on:

	Unit Cost	Cost/ day	Cost/ stay	Quality	Satisfaction RN	other
hi NCI	up	up	down?	no change?	up	down?
lo NCI	(no changes since already lo now)					

Notes: Cost per admission: hi NCI might reduce l.o.s.
Quality: LPNs currently our mainstay and doing a good job
Satisfaction: In the long run hi NCI might improve satisfaction but teams are working smoothly now.

Recommendation: Our NCL of .4 is probably too low, but NCI (r) graph shows this is caused by 6-8 people caring for a few patients. Let's check this out. There's no reason here to change our team size.

2. Repeat this process for each of NAP elements. You will note several things in this process.

   a) Sometimes recommendations for an element taken up later may influence an earlier judgment. Fine. Explain it on the later recommendation, and note the possible shift on the earlier one.

   b) The four coordination elements link closely to your earlier concensus. What you decided about current integration and continuity patterns more or less determines what coordination patterns you need.

   c) Sometimes you are stopped from having a desirable assignment pattern as defined by patient characteristics, by the constraints of nursing resources or organizational support. Note these, and make estimates of the time costs and the dollar costs that would be involved in changing the constraining variables.

   These short-term recommendations call attention to things you may want to try to change, prior to introducing the desirable NAP.

3. After you have completed the analysis for a unit, do the analysis for the other units. This gives you a comparative basis that allows you to check the consistency of your recommendations. It also lets you begin to think about which changes can be made immediately, and which will require longer to achieve (e.g., because they will depend on changes in recruiting practices, or attrition in some types of personnel).

4. Review your overall recommendations:

   a) Consider the financial constraint of the hospital. A severe constraint often means that unit operating costs will be the most important way of measuring cost, that it will be difficult to gain approval for immediate costs increases, and that loss of flexibility may be a severe problem. A normal constraint often means that reduced cost per stay will be given more weight and that well-supported arguments for long-term cost savings will receive attention.

   b) Consider staff availability. If you possibly can, avoid selecting an assignment pattern that will force you to run short-staffed or to face with continual high turnover problems.

   c) Review all your data sources. Some data not specifically used by the connective propositions contained here, may nevertheless be of great importance in your own professional judgment.

   d) Include the specific actions you propose. For example: reduce Aides by four as soon as possible; increase availability and use to standard care protocols; use two-person teams as transition stage; organize special training for RNs; etc.

   e) Estimate the changes in costs, quality, and satisfaction which will result. Express them in measurable terms as much as possible. Indicate when the changes are expected.

5. We strongly encourage you to do this much work *before* you begin discussing these issues with people outside the NAP team. Your close contact with the whole process has given you an ability to be comfortable with the possibility of changes and allows you to discuss possible changes without becoming defensive. That won't be true of people whose contact with the process is minimal. Get a fairly clear idea of what you believe is the right way to proceed before you "go public." There will almost certainly be some changes in your recommendations, but professionals have a right to receive well-considered recommendations, not "mountains of facts . . ." that are still unanalyzed.

6. Discuss the recommendations with Director of Nursing, if Director is not a member of the NAP team.

7. Present recommendations to unit leaders.

   a) Focus on the specific actions recommended and the expected changes they will make in Nursing Assignment elements.

b) Be alert for suggestions that may improve timing or content.

c) Discuss outcome criteria and secure agreement on the measurable changes that can be expected.

8. Develop a complete action recommendation for formal submission and approval. (This can be short by substantiating it with appendixes of documents that already exist; e.g., Recommendations Worksheets and Display Sheets.) By doing this formally, you signal that:

a) Planning is over and it is time for implementation.

b) The administration's formal approval is a public commitment to provide to this plan the organizational support it needs.

9. Take a day off and celebrate. You're done!... until implementation starts tomorrow.

B. NURSING CARE INTEGRATION (NCI)

NCI Range Attributes

In quality,
hi NCI may improve staff members' acceptance of responsibility for care giving and increase the patient's confidence in "having *a* nurse;"
lo NCI may widen the range of specialized skills available to the patient; this is valuable when hi technical complexity, or low standardization and hi variability, makes such skills important.

In cost,
hi NCI minimizes the costs of coordination and by focusing responsibility may minimize costs associated with absenteeism;
lo or medium NCI minimizes training costs and allows more efficient use of specialists and of less skilled personnel.

In personnel satisfaction,
hi NCI satisfies personnel with a strong desire for responsibility;
lo or medium NCI allows a maximum of shared responsibility and avoids the stress of difficult patients being assigned to a single care-giver.

Note:
A hi NCI, almost by definition, eliminates Aides and in many cases LPNs from care giving. In such situations, the per patient cost of care will almost certainly be higher if hi technical requirements of care exist for largely predictable and stable patients. The per patient costs of care will *not* necessarily be higher when complex and unstable patients are cared for by a single care-giver, because the overlapping functions of monitoring, conference, and follow-up activities are eliminated, and length of stay may be reduced due to better care.

NCI Connective Propositions

I. Hi values of NCI are indicated when patient populations have one or more of the following characteristics:

hi instability (but see Ia below)	*Q	11, 18, 86, 211, 229[1]
lo predictability (but see Ia below)	*Q	18, 43, 86, 145, 229, 264
hi complexity of processing (but see Ia below)		18, 208, 264
lo multiple technical requirements	*E	27, 107, 122, 136, 155, 159, 174, 229
pediatric and geriatric patients tend to have hi basic care and technical requirements		56, 159, 174, 251
lo variability	*E	18, 41, 83, 104, 122, 169, 226, 229, 267

A hi NCI is probably less beneficial when patient populations do not have the above characteristics.

Ia. An exception, in which better care may result from a lower NCI, may occur depending on the nature of Nursing Resources and Organizational Support. Particularly with one or more of the following Patient Characteristics:

hi instability

lo predictability

hi complexity of processing

then, medium values of NCI are indicated if Nursing Resources and Organizational Support have one or more of the following characteristics:

Nursing Resources

lo RN/patient ratio		204
lo RN/staff ratio		11, 18, 39, 50, 66, 95, 152, 177, 264
hi RN absenteeism	*	195

---

[1]Numbered abstracts appear in Appendix 1.
Notes: * = important proposition
Q = quality related
E = ease of introduction
$ = cost related

Organizational Support

lo patient care services		126
lo unit support services	E	126

Ib.   When patient population, Nursing Resources, and Organizational Support have one or more of the following characteristics, quality will be less influenced by whether NCI is high or low.

Patient Characteristics

hi predictability	18, 264

Nursing Resources

hi special training programs	66, 240

hi in-service resources

Organizational Support

hi standardization

II.   Hi values of NCI are more readily achieved when Nursing Resources and Organizational Support have the following characteristics:

Nursing Resources

hi RN/staff ratio	*	50, 66, 152
hi preparation ratio		11, 39, 95
lo turnover		53, 152, 195, 207
lo RN absenteeism		195

Organizational Support

hi patient care services	126
hi unit support services	126

A lo or medium value of NCI is more readily achieved when Nursing Resources and Organizational Support do not have the above characteristics.

IIa.   Lo values of NCI are in particular supported by:

hi turnover among RNs and lo turnover among LPNs and Aides	Q

special training for LPNs and Aides

C. CARE MANAGEMENT INTEGRATION (CMI)

CMI Range Attributes

In quality,
   hi CMI encourages focused responsibility and integrated planning of care;
   medium CMI provides necessary professional input to care planning and/or involvement of actual care providers in the care-planning process.

In cost,
   hi CMI minimizes costs of coordination;
   medium CMI minimizes training costs related to maintaining an all-professional staff and allows more efficient use of specialists.

In personnel satisfaction,
   hi CMI satisfies RNs with a strong desire for accountability and lower level staff with a strong desire for clear direction.
   medium CMI satisfies RNs and lower level staff who have a strong desire to share responsibility.

Note:
   Lo CMI has almost nothing to justify its use, except when individual patients with hi complexity and lo predictability are being cared for by narrowly trained and inexperienced personnel in a setting which has lo standardization.

CMI Connective Propositions

I.   Hi values of CMI are indicated when patient populations have one or more of the following characteristics:

hi length of stay (particularly in conjunction with other characteristics on this list)	*Q	33, 37, 154, 168, 197[1]
pediatric patients		268, 90
geriatric patients	Q	41, 171, 172, 174
hi instability	*Q	11, 18, 211, 226, 229
lo predictability (but see Ia below)	*Q	11, 18, 86, 229, 264
hi complexity of processing (but see Ia below)	*	18, 264
hi complex task integration (but see Ia below)	*Q	11, 18, 37, 155, 208, 264

A hi CMI is probably less beneficial when patient populations do not have the above characteristics.

Ia. An exception, in which better care management may result from lower CMI, may occur depending on the nature of Nursing Resources. Particularly with one or more of the following Patient Characteristics:

lo predictability

hi complexity of processing

hi complex task integration

then, medium values of CMI are indicated if Nursing Resources have one or more of the following characteristics:

lo ratio of preparation   *

lo commitment

hi RN turnover

---

[1]Numbered abstracts appear in Appendix 1.

II.   Hi values of CMI are more readily achieved when Nursing Resources and Organizational Support have the following characteristics:

hi RN/patient ratio   172, 195, 202, 204

hi ratio of preparation, or hi standardization   *   18, 33, 39, 47, 55, 152,
                                                                               161, 195, 231, 267

hi RN special training in nursing process   27, 66, 151, 179, 240
and in facilitation of accountability

hi commitment   35

lo turnover   *   53, 152, 195, 248

hi use of clinical nurse specialist (CNS)   18, 25, 264
as care planner; lo use as consultant

lo patient care services[1]   18, 25, 224

---

[1]This proposition really means, "the less outsiders do, the easier it is for nurses to manage the care process."

D. PLAN-DO INTEGRATION (PDI)

PDI Range Attributes

In quality,
hi PDI improves individual or group acceptance of responsibility for care giving and increases the ability to plan with full feedback of results;
lo PDI uses hi-level care management skills where they are most needed.

In cost,
hi PDI may reduce direct patient-care time requirements, and by focusing responsibility may minimize costs associated with absenteeism;
lo PDI minimizes training costs, and allows more efficient use of specialists and less skilled personnel.

In personnel satisfaction,
hi PDI satisfies personnel with a strong desire for responsibility;
lo PDI avoids making highly trained professional nurses perform simple, time-consuming and dependent functions.

Note:
A hi PDI requires a single person *or a single group* to plan and give care. Its value will almost certainly be highest when patients' needs are such that several tasks (for example, patient teaching, bathing, and needs assessment) can be performed simultaneously.

PDI Connective Propositions

I.   Hi values of PDI are indicated when patient populations have one or more of the following characteristics:

hi instability   *Q   11, 18, 86, 211, 226, 229[1]

lo predictability   18, 43, 86, 145, 229, 264, 259

hi complexity of processing   208

hi proportion of females   32, 107

A hi PDI is probably less beneficial when patient populations do not have these characteristics.

Ia. Lo values of PDI are indicated when patient populations have one or more of the following characteristics:

hi multiple technical requirements (but see   *$ 122, 155
Ib below)

hi variability (but see Ib below)   E   18, 33, 37, 41, 69, 83, 86, 104, 122, 123, 226, 229, 267

A lo PDI is probable less beneficial when patient populations do not have these characteristics.

Ib. An exception to Ia, in which the same quality care and improved satisfac tion may result from higher PDI, may occur depending on the nature of Nursing Resources. With one or more of these patient characteristics:

hi multiple technical requirements

hi variability

then, hi values of PDI are indicated if Nursing Resources have one or more of the following characteristics:

hi RN/staff ratio

hi commitment

lo absenteeism

---

[1]Numbered abstracts appear in Appendix 1.

II. Hi values of PDI are more readily achieved when Nursing Resources and Organizational Support have the following characteristics:

Nursing Resources

hi RN/patient ratio   *   175, 195, 202, 204

hi preparation ratio   33, 39, 42, 177, 218, 229, 240

hi RN/staff ratio   *   33, 152

hi special training for RN   45, 53, 66, 179, 240

Organizational Support

hi patient care services   20, 126

hi physical environment   110

hi standardization   259

IIa. Lo values of PDI are appropriate with the following:

Nursing Resources

CNS is only present to plan care   39

lo experience ratio

hi special training for LPN and Aide

E. NURSING CARE CONTINUITY

NCC Range Attributes

In quality,
    hi NCC permits effective teaching, psycho-social support, and monitoring of patients with complex needs;
    lo NCC has no direct quality advantages.

In cost,
    hi NCC may reduce length of stay for certain patients;
    lo NCC considerably increases flexibility in the use of staff and therefore minimizes the required staff/patient ratio.

In satisfaction,
    hi NCC may be satisfying to personnel with a strong desire for responsibility, but may cause boredom (from non-challenging patients) on the one hand, and excessive stress (from demanding, difficult, or terminal patients) on the other.

Note:
Hi NCC advantages are specific to certain patients. An optimum assignment pattern will provide hi NCC for those patients and yet remain flexible for other patients in the continuity of their nursing care assignments.

NCC Connective Propositions

I.   Hi values of NCC are indicated when patients have one or more of the following characteristics:

lo length of stay	E	33, 37, 154, 267[1]
geriatric patients	Q	41, 172, 174
lo predictability	Q	18, 43, 86, 145, 229, 264
hi complexity of task integration	*Q	11, 155
hi multiple learning requirements	*Q	31, 52, 66
lo multiple technical requirements	E	155

A hi NCC is probably less beneficial when patients do not have the above characteristics.

II.   Hi values of NCC are more readily achieved when Nursing Resources and Organizational Support have the following characteristics:

Nursing Resources

hi RN/staff ratio		42, 104
lo absenteeism (all staff)		
hi commitment	*	190

Organizational Support

permanent shifts		
lo staffing instability	*	
lo part-time ratio		

---

[1] Numbered abstracts appear in Appendix 1.

F. CARE MANAGEMENT CONTINUITY (CMC)

CMC Range Attributes

In quality,

it is possible to achieve appropriate levels of Care Management Continuity and not achieve desired results. In general, hi CMC facilitates meeting hi learning needs and complex care needs, but will do neither unless Care Management Integration (CMI) is hi and Nursing Coordination (NC) is matched with it. Hi CMC can benefit patients whose care needs are predictable or unpredictable, but when such needs are highly unpredictable expert level competence will be required for hi CMC to be effective.

lo CMC has no direct quality advantages, but because lo CMC permits more flexible use of staff it should be accepted, unless the benefits and the possibility of hi CMC are clear. A partial way of testing the importance of having hi CMC is to ask, "How many days sooner would this patient be ready for discharge if an experienced and expert nurse had full and continuous responsibility for his care?"

In cost,

hi CMC may reduce length of stay for some patients;
lo CMC permits more flexible use of staff.

In personnel satisfaction,

hi CMC moves toward full accountability for a patient's care, but may also lead to sharp status distinctions among nurses that will increase dissatisfactions among others on the nursing staff.

CMC across settings (CMCt):

Care management continuity across settings (CMCt) represents an approach to defining assignment patterns which transcends the patient unit structure. Therefore it suggests a radical departure from common nursing structures. From the point of view of the unit, hi CMCt means the addition of a professional quite parallel to the physician, who makes nursing diagnosis and writes nursing orders that unit nursing personnel follow. From the point of view of the unit, all nursing functions, both care and cure, become "dependent" functions.

An obvious source of such professional care managers are unit nursing personnel, though they are not the only source. A nursing department is well advised not to introduce hi CMCt unless all other parts of the assignment pattern have been thought through and clearly established. In that setting, patients with specific characteristics may benefit significantly from hi CMCt.

CMC Connective Propositions

I.   Hi CMC *within the unit* is indicated when patients have one or more of the following characteristics:

pediatric patients (especially toddlers)		187[1]
geriatric patients (over age 65)		41, 171, 172
lo instability	*	33, 37, 69, 123, 155, 171
hi complexity of processing		208
hi complex task integration		11, 37, 155
hi multiple learning needs	*Q	31, 52, 66

Hi CMC is probably less beneficial when patient populations do not have these characteristics.

Ia.   When patient characteristics indicate one or more of the following:

hi complexity of processing,

hi complex task integration,

lo predictability,

then, a hi preparation ratio is desirable to   11, 18, 86, 145, 229, 264
provide hi CMC.

II.   Hi values of CMC are more readily achieved when the variables below have the characteristics specified:

Patient Characteristics and Nursing Coordination

hi predictability	E	123, 127
nursing coordination by autonomy	E	

Nursing Resources and Organizational Support

hi RN/staff ratio	*	154, 202, 240, 266
hi use of CNS as care giver or consultant		39

---

[1]Numbered abstracts appear in Appendix 1.

lo part-time ratio

special RN training in nursing process and in   *   27, 45, 56, 66, 179, 240
facilitation of accountability

lo RN absenteeism

hi standardization

III.   Care Management Continuity *across settings* (CMCt) is indicated when patients and organizational support have one or more of the following characteristics:

lo length of stay   *   154, 168, 197

lo instability   154, 168, 181, 226, 267

hi predictability   116, 181

hi standardization   225

IIIa.   Hi values of CMCt are more readily achieved when:

Other elements of the Nursing Assignment Pattern are clearly defined and include a hi CMI and CMC and proactive Care-Cure and Patient Services Coordination.

MSN and BSN prepared nurses are available   39, 267
to implement CMC across settings.

G. NURSING COORDINATION (NC)

NC Range Attributes

In quality,
nursing coordination has no simple relation to quality. The key is to match methods of coordinating patient care with the selected levels of the integration elements (NCI, CMI, PDI).

In cost,
coordination by autonomy requires more costly personnel, but permits them to spend less time coordinating activities. Consultation and hierarchy allow the use of less costly personnel, with consultation having the highest coordination time requirement.

In satisfaction,
coordination by hierarchy is least likely to provide hi levels of satisfaction. Consultation can lead to highest interpersonal satisfaction, often a decisive factor in overall satisfaction.

NC Connective Propositions

I. Hi values of NCI favor NC by autonomy.

                                                    11, 27, 151[1]

Ia. Hi values of PDI favor NC by autonomy or consultation.

                            *   41, 169, 171, 267

Ib. Hi values of CMI favor NC by autonomy or hierarchy.

                                                    123, 167

Ic. With hi CMCt, NC is by hierarchy or consultation.

                                                    154, 267

Id. Only hierarchical or consultative coordination are feasible when a unit has a significant number of LPNs and Aides.

                            *   25, 67, 69, 118

II. The presence of high levels of standardization allows the use of autonomous coordination by a wider range of professional personnel, and reduces the need for and advantages of consultative coordination.

                            *$ 41, 123, 169

IIa. Lo staff stability in a unit workforce, whether due to absenteeism, turnover, or staff instability, makes NC by autonomy least feasible and by hierarchy most feasible.

IIb. Special training programs and strong in-service capability allow a choice among NC alternatives.

IIc. Hi physician-nurse collegiality, support services, and patient services all facilitate NC by autonomy; their absence favors coordination by hierarchy.

                                                    25, 51, 106, 179

---

[1]Numbered abstracts appear in Appendix 1.

H. CARE-CURE COORDINATION (CCC) AND PATIENT SERVICES COORDINATION (PSC)

CCC and PSC Range Attributes

In quality,
   proactive coordination provides leadership from the professional closest to the patient.

In cost,
   proactive coordination is often time-consuming and its use may increase the number of RN hours required per patient.

In satisfaction,
   proactive coordination satisfies nurses with strong commitments to professional patient care.

Note:
   Proactive coordination provides a leading role for the nurse (or head nurse) in relating to physicians and other health care professionals. Accordingly, it requires adequate support services, high competence in nurses, and respect and support from the professionals being coordinated, as well as the types of patient needs which make its relevance clear. The absence of any of these conditions suggests that efforts to improve the supporting conditions should be made before major attempts to introduce proactive nursing are undertaken.

CCC and PSC Connective Propositions

I.   Proactive coordination is indicated when patient populations have the following characteristics:

hi instability   *Q   11, 33, 37, 128, 208[1]

hi variability (nurse proactive especially indicated)

hi complexity of processing (nurse proactive   208
especially indicated)

hi complex task integration (nurse proactive   11, 155
especially indicated)

hi multiple coordination requirements   *   11, 161, 259, 268

Pediatric patients (nurse proactive PSC
especially indicated)

Proactive coordination is probably less beneficial when patient populations do not have these characteristics.

II. Proactive coordination is more easily achieved under the following conditions:

Nursing Assignment Elements

hi CMI   33, 37

hi PDI

hi CMC

Patient Characteristics

hi predictability   11, 33, 37, 128, 155, 180

Nursing Resources

hi RN/patient ratio   240, 266, 268

hi RN/staff ratio   49, 69, 161, 240

special training for RNs in nursing process   45, 47, 53, 240
and leadership

hi commitment

[1]Numbered abstracts appear in Appendix 1.

Organizational Resources

hi physician-nurse communication (for proactive CCC)		71, 161
hi physician-nurse collegiality (for proactive CCC)	*	18, 48, 71
hi patient care services (for proactive PSC)		21, 51, 152
lo physician presence	*	220
hi standardization		

I. INTER-SHIFT COORDINATION (ISC)

ISC Range Attributes

In quality,
ISC by integrated patient record or specially developed care plan provides continuity in care to patients with complex needs;
ISC by report and standard care plans does the same for patients with less complex needs.

In cost,
ISC by integrated patient record or specially developed care plan requires hi-level resources and is therefore more costly than ISC by report and standard care plans.

In satisfaction,
ISC by integrated patient record or specially developed care plan satisfies nurses with a strong desire for accountability, but may be less satisfying to nurses who do not share in the care planning.

ISC Connective Propositions

I. Variables which suggest hi values for NCC and CMC favor ISC by integrated patient record or specially developed care plan. Variables which suggest low values of NCC and CMC favor ISC by report and standard care protocols or plans.

$$11, 31, 37, 41, 56, 66,$$
$$69, 123, 155, 171, 172,$$
$$174[1]$$

Ia. With hi levels of CMCt, ISC by integrated patient record or specially developed care plan is required.

$$33, 37, 69, 123, 155, 157$$

II. Hi levels of standardization and predictability favor ISC by report and standard care protocols or plans.

$$11, 18, 86, 145, 229, 264$$

III. ISC by integrated patient record or specially developed care plan is more readily achieved when Nursing Resources and Organizational Support have one or more of the following characteristics:

Nursing Resources

hi preparation ratio

hi RN/patient ratio

hi RN/staff ratio

special training in documentation, nursing   45, 47, 53, 66, 69, 151,
process, and leadership   179, 240

Organizational Support

hi physician-nurse collegiality

hi evening/night shift patient care services

---

[1]Numbered abstracts appear in Appendix 1.

J. COST IMPLICATIONS OF CHANGES IN NURSING ASSIGNMENT ELEMENTS

There is relatively little in the literature that provides good data on the cost implications of various elements in the nursing assignment pattern. This is not surprising, given the strong emphasis on quality which characterizes the literature, but it is not very helpful either. We have provided the following material on the cost implications of nursing assignment changes as a rough guide, to help you make estimates of cost effects. It rests in part on observations made during the demonstration project in which the instrumentation in this manual was developed, but has no other empirical foundation.

"Cost implications" is of course an imprecise term. Do we mean cost per stay (cost per admission)? Cost per patient day? If you reduce length of stay, cost per stay will go down, but because you are probably eliminating days of stay with few services, cost per day will go up. There is a third cost concept, unit operating costs, and this way of viewing costs is what is reflected on monthly operating statements. We've already suggested in Section IV G ways of getting measures of what will happen to these costs, but the problem is that you can't wait for that; you have to make assumptions *now* about their effects.

We have put together a chart (Figure VI:3) that will be of some help to you. It includes some of the most significant influences on cost which may be altered by a change in assignment pattern:

1. Length of stay. There is growing evidence that nursing care can influence the amount of hospitalization needed by some patients, sometimes dramatically. For this to actually influence costs, physicians must of course be willing to adjust their discharge decisions accordingly. A reduction in length of stay reduces cost per stay, increases cost per day, and reduces unit operating costs unless occupancy increases.

2. Staff numbers. Adjusting elements in the assignment pattern may increase or decrease the number of nursing staff required. This has a direct effect on cost per stay, cost per day, and unit operating costs.

3. Staff levels. Probably the most obvious effect of changing the assignment pattern is on changing the level (RN, LPN, Aide) of staffing required. When there are very small differentials in salary, the effect may be trivial. But if there are large salary differentials, for example an Aide costing one-half the amount of an RN, then changes in staff levels become important.

A change in staff level can affect all three cost measures: cost per stay, cost per day, and unit operating costs.

4. Training requirements. Costs which may be incurred by having to spend more time increasing the skills of your staff. Remember these are usually "double" costs, the costs of paying the trainers, and the costs of "covering" the trainees on the unit. (If you don't need to cover them, are you overstaffed?) Training effects all three cost measures.

5. Loss of flexibility. Some changes in assignment patterns make it more difficult to fully utilize staff (e.g., not being able to pull nurses, reschedule patient assignments, adjust for absenteeism, etc.). This is particularly true for the continuity elements, because high continuity reduces your ability to shift staff in response to changing patient needs or available personnel. Such loss of flexibility effects all three cost measures.

A general rule: Be very realistic when you are estimating cost effects. This whole study can help establish or reaffirm nursing personnel as rational, clear-headed decision makers. A year or two years from now these decisions can come back to haunt you if they are based on foolish optimism rather than careful assessments.

Figure VI:3
Probable Cost Implications of Increases in NAP Elements

An increase in a NAP element may affect the following variables, and thus cause an
increase (+) or decrease (–), or no change (0) in costs.

	Length of Stay	Staff Numbers	Staff Levels	Training Requirements	Loss of Flexibility
↑ NCI	–	–	+	+	+
↑ CMI	0	–	+	+	+
↑ PDI	–	–	++	++	+
↑ NCC	–	+	+	0	++
↑ CMC	––	+	0	0	++
(autonomy) NC	0	–	+	0	–
CCC, (proactive) PSC	–	0	+	+	–
ISC	––	0	–	+	+

Short-stay patients reduce the impact of these savings.	Standardized care protocols reduce the impact of these costs. High RN/LPN/Aide differentials increase the impact of these costs.	Few part-time staff and low turnover reduce the impact of these costs.	High proportion of part-time staff and stable census reduce the impact of these costs.

KEY:
- ++ = Significant cost increase
- + = Some cost increase
- 0 = No cost change
- – = Some cost decrease
- –– = Significant cost decrease

VII
APPENDIXES

Appendix 1

AN ANNOTATED BIBLIOGRAPHY ON NURSING ASSIGNMENT DECISIONS

Compiled and edited by
Joanne Shultz Beckman

This bibliography is the product of an 18-month project, "Defining Appropriate Nursing Assignment Patterns," conducted by faculty and staff of the Bureau of Hospital Administration, University of Michigan and funded by the W. K. Kellogg Foundation of Battle Creek, Michigan. The literature review which formed the basis of this compilation covered the years 1960 through 1976 and utilized a variety of sources for searches of the literature, in particular three excellent reviews:

Aydelotte, M. *Nursing staffing methodology: A review and critique of selected literature.* U.S. Dept. of Health, Education, and Welfare, Pub. No. (NIH) 73–433, January 1973.

Georgopoulos, B. S. *Hospital organization research: Review and source book.* Philadelphia: W. B. Saunders Co., 1974.

Medicus Systems Corporation. *A review and evaluation of nursing productivity. Vol. I and II. Conference Proceedings and Final Report.* The Corporation, October 1975, January 1976.

Articles relevant to decisions on nursing assignment patterns were selected and annotated. On the basis of the literature review, guidelines to selecting or changing assignment patterns were developed: these "connective propositions" discussed in Section VI of this manual are referenced to the numbered entries here.

Several abbreviations are used to indicate the type of information in the article and its relevance to assignment decisions. Four topic areas were defined in the project as having particular influence on the appropriateness of an assignment pattern: these were (1) the current assignment pattern in use on a unit, (2) the characteristics of patients on the unit, (3) the nursing resources available to the unit, and (4) the organizational support systems available. The following abbreviations are used as indexes at the right hand side of each citation to facilitate location of articles according to topic and type of study described:

Nursing assignment pattern:	NAP:
total patient care	TPC
team nursing	TM
primary nursing	PN
functional nursing	FN
case assignment	CS
Patient characteristics:	PC
Nursing resources:	NR
Organizational support:	OS
Empirical study:	*
Report of implementation:	+

For example, an article indexed as:

NAP*: PN, TM

is an empirical study of primary and team nursing assignment patterns:

NAP⁺: PN

is a report of the implementation of primary nursing on a unit;

NAP, PC

is a discussion of assignment patterns in general and also describes characteristics of the patient populations under consideration.

Whenever possible, we have provided sufficient information for you to obtain copies of the article. To acquire documents available from University Microfilms International, all relevant facts especially the full document number must be included.

Grateful acknowledgment is made to the following copyright owners for permission to reprint abstracts appearing in this Appendix:

Administrative Science Quarterly (059, 208)
Appleton-Century-Crofts (237)
Hospital Research and Educational Trust (147)
Journal of Nursing Administration (049, 173, 270, 272)
W. K. Kellogg Foundation (185)
C. V. Mosby Company (080, 081)
University Microfilms International (005, 058, 061)
Western Interstate Commission for Higher Education (008, 030, 076, 116, 136)
John Wiley & Sons, Inc. (040)

The production of this bibliography involved the efforts of many people. The following persons made major contributions to the literature review and annotations; their initials appear at the end of annotations they prepared:

Joanne S. Beckman, R.N., M.S.
Jacqueline Clinton, R.N., M.A.
Carolyn Keever, R.N., M.P.H.
Jennifer P. Kelley, B.A.
Barbara Kennison, R.N., M.S.
Cynthia A. Leatherman, R.N., M.S.

Larry McCreery cheerfully typed the entire final manuscript. Tom Gunderson, Emma Williams, and Allison Stieber assisted in typing, editing, or proofreading. Fred Munson and Barbara Horn provided much appreciated support and direction to the effort. The combined contributions of all made compiling and editing this bibliography an easy and pleasant task.

References

001   PC

Abdellah, F., & Levine, E. *Better patient care through nursing research*. London: The Macmillan Company, 1965.

Presents basic concepts of research in nursing, particularly those concerned with patient care. Overview of research process and citations of applications of research to nursing and patient care situations. Chapter 12, pp. 446–475, provides excellent comments and review of patient classification methods. Chapters 13 and 14 review descriptive and explanatory studies in nursing and patient care. (Significant studies are referenced separately.) (JB)

002   NR, PC, NAP

Abdellah, F. G., Meyer, B., & Roberts, H. Nursing patterns vary in progressive care. *The Modern Hospital*. August 1960, 95(2): 85–91.

Purpose of the study was to provide information relative to the nurse staffing practices of non-federal general hospitals that had established one or more progressive care elements. The survey revealed that most hospitals had organized only one of the progressive patient care elements—an intensive care area. The results of 71 ICUs were compared. Data revealed a tremendous amount of variation in staffing patterns. The variability was attributed, at least in part, to: (1) the utilization of nonprofessional nurses, (2) the size of the facility, (3) the type of patient cared for, and (4) the layout of the facility. The nurse staffing experiences of three hospitals whose predominant organizational pattern was progressive patient care are presented in detail; an additional hospital with an ICU is also described. (BK)

003   NR, OS

Abstracts of Health Care Management Studies. Published quarterly by Health Administration Press for the Cooperative Information Center for Health Care Management Studies, The University of Michigan, Ann Arbor, Mich. 48109.

An international journal with abstracts of studies of management, planning, and public policy related to the delivery of health care. Purposes of the Information Center are to find new and noncirculated studies, assemble current information, and make new studies readily available. Formerly titled *Abstracts of Hospital Management Studies*. (JB)

004   PC, NR, NAP⁺:CS

Alfano, G. J. The Loeb Center for nursing and rehabilitation: A professional approach to nursing. *Nursing Clinics of North America*. September 1969, 4:487.

This article describes the general staffing plan at Loeb Center, lines of authority and a progress report after six years of implementing the case method. High satisfaction of nurses, other professionals, and clients, lower costs and readmission rates compared to other hospitals are reported. Rehabilitation patients. (JC)

005   NR, NAP

Allison, R. F. *The role of the nurses' aide*. (Doctoral dissertation, University of Michigan, 1972) Ann Arbor, Mich.: University Microfilms International, No. 73–11,030.

The focus of this study is the role of the nurses' aide and the role system in which it is embedded. The study includes a history and theory of the development of hospitals and such health professional roles as physicians, professional nurses, licensed practical nurses, and nurses' aides. The empirical case study involved 80 nurses' aides, 29 RNs and 34 LPNs from a medium-size general hospital. The normative role sent to the aide and the behavioral role the aide perceives herself to be performing were measured separately and compared. The behavior reported by aides substantially conformed to the expectations of the health professional determined to be the most significant other to the aide—the RN. Nurses (RNs) agreed on the "team" role for aides, while aides tended to see themselves more autonomously as the patient's helper. Some of the findings contradict statements in the literature as to the degree of supervision of aides. (Author's abstract adapted)

006   PC, NR, OS

American Nurses' Association, Committee on Nursing Services. *Statement on nursing staff requirements for in-patient health care services*. New York: The Association, 1967.

This statement outlines criteria for developing staffing patterns for inpatient care services suited to the individual needs of particular units. It outlines the factors, policies, and procedures to be considered in determining requirements. (From *Planning for Nursing Needs and Resources,* DHEW Pub. No. (NIH) 72-87, p. 135, April 1972)

007 NAP⁺: PN

Anderson, M. Primary nursing in day-by-day practice. *American Journal of Nursing.* May 1976, 76(5):802–805.

A conversational how-to article describing ways to ease the transition and reduce the irritants a nursing service department may encounter in switching over from traditional nurse staffing to primary nursing. The author has been a staff nurse and an inservice nurse on a station where primary nursing was practiced at the University of Minnesota Hospitals, Minneapolis. Problems associated with the system of primary nursing and the role of the head nurse in particular, are discussed. (CAL)

008 PC

Anderson, R. S. Two decades of change in obstetrical practices in hospitals in King County. (Unpublished master's thesis, University of Washington, School of Nursing, 1973).

This descriptive study surveyed the changes that have occurred and the rate of change in obstetrical department practices in the hospitals in King County between the years of 1952 and 1972. The study was primarily concerned with those changes in practice brought about by consumer influence. Data were collected by means of a factual questionnaire completed by the nursing staffs of the obstetrical departments. Analysis of the data indicated an exponential rate of change occurred with the greatest increase in the acceptance of more family-centered and individualized maternity care in the period after 1967. There was an increase in practices allowing the mother more individual choice in the conduct of her labor, delivery and postpartum period, greater father participation, an increase in mother-baby interaction, and father-baby interaction, and more emphasis on parental education for childbirth and baby care. (Abstract adapted from Western Interstate

Commission on Higher Education in Nursing, *Newly Initiated and Completed Research,* Vol. 11, December 1975).

009 NAP: CS, PN

Arnsdorf, M. B. Perceptions of primary nursing in a family-centered care setting. *Nursing Administration Quarterly.* Winter 1977, 1(2):97–105.

This article offers information on the evaluation of "family-centered nursing." Components of this type of nursing include: (1) caseload assignment, (2) patient and family assessment, (3) accountability and responsibility for the RN, (4) care-giver to care-giver communication, interdepartmental collaboration, and discharge planning and follow-through. The author identifies family involvement in the patient's care, and an additional component of interdepartmental collaboration as the major marks of difference between this system and that described by Ciske. Basic responsibilities of the nurse under this pattern included: (1) prehospitalization interviewing, (2) admitting procedure and initial assessment, (3) maintaining care for the patient in-house *while on duty,* (4) ensuring implementation of discharge, (5) caring for the patient following discharge, and (6) maintaining continuity of care during in-house transfer. (JC)

010 PC, NAP⁺:TM

Auld, M. G. Team nursing in a maternity hospital. *International Journal of Nursing Studies,* 1970, 7(2): 57–66.

Description of a nine-month experiment in a British maternity hospital to implement team nursing on one floor. Team nursing was viewed as a means to alleviate the depersonalization of patients when the staff is assigned to one of several areas of maternity care, either prenatal, postnatal, labor ward or nursery, "inevitably leading the nurse to focus her attention on the area of work rather than on specific individuals." Among the observed outcomes were better use of skills, increased time with patients, increased staff-patient satisfaction, and decreased absenteeism and turnover. The major criticism of those nurses who did not like team nursing was inadequate preparation for implementation of the method. (CAL)

011   NAP, NR, OS

Aure, B. & Schneider, J. M. Transforming a community hospital nursing service into a regional center. *Nursing Clinics of North America,* June 1975, 10(2): 275–291.

Description of the transformation of a traditional community hospital obstetric service into a perinatal center, including changes in administration, addition of clinical specialists and nurse clinicians, upgrading and changing care practices. This article describes the impact of the change on a traditional maternity nursing service. The change was based on the premise that nursing is a keystone to successful patient outcomes and is on a peer level with medicine. The collaboration of nurses and physicians as planners and administrators of this program, with strong administrative support and consistent expectations of staff with concomitant help, support, and educational input was effective in upgrading care and changing nursing behavior. Continuing problems included communication between units and personnel. (JB)

012

Aydelotte, M. K. The use of patient welfare as a criterion measure. *Nursing Research,* Winter 1962, 2(1): 10–14. (See #016.)

Study was done to determine if an increase in the amount and quality of nursing care would produce improvements in patient welfare. This was tested in two ways: (1) increasing size of ward nursing staff, and (2) introducing an educational program to increase the amount and quality of nursing care. A total of five experiments were conducted. Results revealed that increasing staff and/or inservice education did not produce any noticeable improvement in patient welfare. The main focus of this paper is restricted to a general description/discussion and defense of patient welfare measures used. (BK)

013   NR, OS

Aydelotte, M. K. *Survey of hospital nursing services.* New York: National League for Nursing, 1968.

This is a report of a questionnaire survey of 93 items pertaining to the current status of nursing service activities in 1,172 short-term, general, nonfederal, nonpsychiatric hospitals of all sizes. The survey, conducted in 1964, was intended to stimulate hospital nursing services to examine their status as a basis for implementing the criteria for effective nursing service developed by the National League for Nursing. Survey findings highlighted in the report include: nursing services' continuity for other services; limited in-service education programs; a variety of hospital educational programs; and the characteristics and activities of directors of nursing service. Survey findings point to needed changes in the organization and administration of nursing services and improved leadership for its administration. (Abstract from *Planning for Nursing Needs and Resources.* DHEW Pub. No. (NIH) 72–87 App. 2, p. 158, April 1972) (CAL)

014   NAP, NR

Aydelotte, M. K. *Nursing staffing methodology: A review and critique of selected literature.* DHEW Pub. No. (NIH) 73–433, January 1973. (See also #163)

This excellent source contains detailed, critical assessments of nearly 200 major methodological studies in the area of nurse staffing and a comprehensive bibliography of more than 1,000 staffing studies. In addition, it presents an historical development of nurse staffing studies, provides a framework for classifying staffing methodology, and contains a detailed glossary of terms used in staffing research. Useful to all concerned with problems of nurse staffing. A companion volume is DHEW, Division of Nursing, *Research on Nurse Staffing in Hospitals: Report of the Conference,* May 1972. (Adapted from Foreword) (JB)

015   NR

Aydelotte, M. K. Staffing for quality care. In Warstler, M. E. (ed.) *Staffing: A Journal of Nursing Administration Reader.* Wakefield, Mass.: Contemporary Publishing, Inc., 1974. (See #263)

Excellent discussion of the development of a staffing program. Four elements of a staffing program are defined and discussed: (1) identification of the quality of the product to be rendered to the client, (2) prediction of the number and kind of personnel needed to produce the volume and quality of care required, (3) selection and arrangement of the nursing staff in specific configurations and the development of assignment patterns for the staff required 24 hours per day, 7 days per week, and (4) evaluation of the effectiveness of staff's product (nursing care) upon the patient population to whom it is rendered. (JB)

016   NAP, NR*, OS*

Aydelotte, M. K. & Tener, M. *An investigation of the relation between nursing activity and patient welfare.* Iowa City: University of Iowa, 1960.

The purpose of this study, which included five experimental variations, was to test the assumption that increases in the amount or quality of nursing care will produce improvements in patient welfare. This was tested by increasing the size of a ward nursing staff and by introducing an in-service educational program designed to increase the amount and quality of the nursing care given by a ward staff. Neither incrementing staff nor the educational program resulted in increases in patient welfare. The educational program appeared to include team nursing concepts. (JB)

017   OS

Ayers, R., Bishop, R. & Moss, F. An experiment in nursing service reorganization. *American Journal of Nursing.* April 1969, 783–786.

This paper describes the departure from a traditional ladder-type organizational structure where advancement and salary increase was based on "status," to an organizational structure that allowed advancement both horizontally and vertically based on nurses' professional competencies and interests. (BK)

018   PC, NR, OS

Backscheider, J. The clinical nursing specialist as practitioner. *Nursing Forum.* 1971, 10(4): 359–377.

Summary of functions of the CNS, from the author's observations and interviews with 25 practicing clinical specialists. Sections of the article describe the CNS role, common features in CNS positions and approaches, educational requirements, problems in implementing the new roles, and implications for the health care system and nursing education. (JB)

019   NR, OS

Baden, C. & Huebosch, J. A. Staffing and staff relations in coronary care units. *Nursing Clinics of North America.* December 1969, 4(4): 573–584.

These authors state that the successful operation of a coronary care unit requires adequately trained professional and supportive nonprofessional personnel. A CCU operates as an independent social system that requires: (1) maintenance of staff through recruitment, (2) provision for initial and ongoing education, and (3) allocation and precise definition of roles, duties, and responsibilities. Role conflict is discussed with the view that interaction of diverse personalities generate conflict; conflicts may disrupt the social system or they may stimulate creative innovations and beneficial change. (JC)

020   NR, OS

Baker, C. & Kramer, M. To define or not to define: The role of the clinical specialist. *Nursing Forum.* 1970, 9(1): 41–55.

An interview survey of directors of nursing in 37 medical centers in the United States was done to ascertain the extent of utilization of the CNS, the scope of the functions of this role, and the implications for patient care and organizational structure. Baccalaureate staff nurses in the same centers were also interviewed. Authors conclude that clear performance and role expectations must exist in both the formal and informal systems within which the CNS operates. Recommendations are given. (JB)

021 NAP⁺:PN

Bakke, K. Primary nursing: Perceptions of a staff nurse. *American Journal of Nursing.* August 1974, 74(8):1432–1434.

This article describes a staff nurse's perceptions of what it is like day-to-day for nurses and patients on a unit where nurses are assigned as primary nurses. Described is the direct referral and communication between nurses and other services, i.e., dietary, occupational therapy, ministers, physical therapy, etc. Author cites "continuity of care" as a major focus of primary nursing. She contends that it is much more difficult to attain this with team nursing, where each member approaches the patient with a task in mind. If some problem is expressed to any one member of a team, is it followed through? Does a team member take responsibility or does the patient's concern get lost in the shuffle? Does the patient know to whom he can relate specific information? Primary nursing is defined as a system in which one nurse gives "total patient care" and is responsible on a 24-hour basis. (JC)

022 NAP:CS, FN, TM

Barabas, M. H. *Contemporary head nursing.* New York: The Macmillan Company, 1962.

This volume is essentially a "how to" book for the purpose of orienting a head nurse to the hospital organizational structure and problems in unit management. Chapter 5 includes a discussion on the advantages and disadvantages of three "conventional" methods of nurse assignment patterns: case method, functional method, and team method. (JC)

023 OS

Barham, V. A patient-oriented nursing system starting as an inter-disciplinary project on the postsurgical service. *Journal of Nursing Administration.* February 1976, 6(2):40.

A patient-oriented nursing service was achieved on a surgical unit by concentrating the equipment for patient care at the bedside and by streamlining forms for the documentation of care, by making appropriate use of pharmacists' expertise, and by involving affected personnel in the process and its goals. (JB)

024 PC, NR

Barr, A., Moores, B. & Rhys-Hearn, C. A review of the various methods of measuring the dependency of patients on nursing staff. *International Journal of Nursing Studies.* August 1973, 10(3):195–208.

This informative article chronologically reviews and contrasts various methods of determining patient dependency and staff needs. A summary table of methods is included. Differences in approach are highlighted. (JC)

025 NR, OS

Barrett, J. Administrative factors in development of new nursing practice roles. *Journal of Nursing Administration.* July-August 1971, 25–29.

The purpose of this article was not to discuss new roles, as such, but to look at the contingencies which may spell the difference between lasting success, temporary success, or lack of success in the development of a new nursing practice role. The author uses the clinical nursing specialist role and factors related to implementation of this role as an illustration. (JC)

026 NR, OS, NAP⁺:TM

Bauer, A. B. *An experimental in-service program for implementing team nursing.* New York: National League for Nursing, 1966.

Study of an in-service program for preparing nursing personnel for a change from functional to team nursing analyzes reports of nursing personnel before change, during process of change, and after team nursing was inaugurated in a 40-bed medical unit of a large general hospital where the physical set up seemed appropriate for the use of team nursing. Group-centered activity was employed to promote favorable psychological atmosphere. Orientation conferences were set up for both professional and nonprofessional members of the nursing staff. Outlines of these conferences and of the function of key members of the team are included in the Appendix. Results of the change to team nursing after this preparation were favorably reported by both patients and team members. (Adapted from *Abstracts of Hospital Management Studies,* June 1968, IV:166.)

027   PC, NR, OS, NAP:TPC

Beckman, J. & Kever, C. Interviews at Bottsford Hospital, Detroit. Personal communication, 1977.

Interviews with nursing and in-service education personnel; description of total patient care and support systems in a local hospital. (JB)

028   NR

Behling, O. C. & Kosmo, R. Reducing nursing turnover. *Hospitals.* February 1, 1971, 45(3): 124–126.

This article indicated that some factors causing nursing turnover are beyond the control of the administrator. Turnover among professional staff nurses is a major problem for hospital and nursing administrators. Much effort in the past has been devoted to reducing the sources of job dissatisfaction on the assumption that job dissatisfaction is a major source of nursing turnover. The notion that highly satisfied nurses are less likely to leave a hospital is logically sound and supported by empirical evidence. Yet job dissatisfaction is not the only source of turnover. The highly satisfied nurse who does leave illustrates turnover caused by a factor other than dissatisfaction. Much turnover is associated with personal and demographic factors that are beyond the control of the administrator. (JC)

029   NR, OS

Bergman, R. Nursing manpower: Issues and trends. *Journal of Nursing Administration.* May 1975, 5(4):21–25.

The current concern over nursing manpower stems from today's so-called shortage, which may be real or due to poor management of existing personnel. Long-range planning is the basis for developing a viable supply-need balance. The critical points in manpower planning are: on the supply side—production, effective use of personnel, and reduction of attrition in the labor force; on the need side—development of appropriate services for the real

needs of the population. Notes problems when support services are inadequate; discusses history of determining levels of personnel needed for each unit. (JB)

030   PC*

Berry, D. M. *An inpatient classification system for nursing service staffing decisions.* (Doctoral dissertation, University of Arizona, 1974.)

Describes a patient classification tool which was developed and tested for reliability and validity for the clinical services of medicine, surgery, intensive care, pediatrics, orthopedics, and obstetrics. It contains five empirically significant dimensions of patient need for nursing care: physical care, emotional, medical regime, teaching, and observations needs. The items and subitems are internally consistent. (Abstract adapted from Western Interstate Commission for Higher Education in Nursing, *Newly Initiated and Completed Research,* Vol. 11, December 1975.)

031   NR, NAP[+]:PN

Bolder, J. NAQ forum: Primary nursing: Why not? *Nursing Administration Quarterly.* Winter 1977, 1(2):79–82.

This is a series of short articles written by different authors about primary nursing. Pertinent articles will be abstracted separately. Primary nursing is viewed by Bolder as a philosophy rather than a patient assignment pattern. This article describes a project of implementing and evaluating primary nursing in one hospital. Primary nursing facilitated the nursing process and teaching-learning activities. The transition was different for LPNs and aides. (JC)

032   PC*

Bouchard, R. E. *An investigation of total nursing needs in two general hospitals and one cancer hospital as a basis for determining the kind and amount of nursing personnel necessary to meet these needs.* (Doctoral dissertation, New York University, 1959) Ann Arbor, Mich.: University Microfilms International, No. 60–1120.

An investigation of the total nursing needs in

two general hospitals and one cancer hospital was done in order to determine the kind and amount of nursing personnel required to meet these needs. A pilot study was used to develop a checklist of patients' nursing needs and behaviors; a patient questionnaire was also used. Data were collected daily on nursing needs, medications used, treatments given, and the time necessary to perform them. Data was coded by age, sex, and diagnosis and was analyzed by t-test and chi square. Patients on medical services in the three hospitals were the subjects, and were comparable in age, race, religion, and socio-economic status. Patients had needs in all areas, including physiological, therapeutic, psychological, sociological, spiritual, basic individual, and physical care. Needs varied with different patients in all three hospitals. Regardless of diagnosis, needs differed significantly according to sex, with needs of female patients greater and more frequent in all areas. Needs also differed significantly according to diagnosis, with cancer patients having greater and more frequent needs in most areas than noncancer patients. No apparent difference was present in the variety of needs exhibited by patients according to sex or diagnosis. Cancer patients had more specialized and greater volume of treatments than noncancer patients. A staffing pattern was proposed: leadership of a team of nursing personnel by a professional (baccalaureate degree) nurse. The author notes the staffing pattern; would not be the same for all hospitals. The study concludes that time, in addition to physical care time, must be allocated if the total nursing needs of the patient are to be met, and that continuous reevaluation of needs as they change from day to day is necessary. (JB)

033   NR, NAP⁺:PN

Bowar-Ferres, S. Loeb Center and its philosophy of nursing. *American Journal of Nursing.* May 1975, 75(5):810–815.

A description of the philosophy of care at Loeb where patients receive skilled, individualized care at their selected pace and manner, nurses practice with a high degree of satisfaction and challenge, and the community benefits from lowered health care costs and from shorter hospitalization. For nearly 12 years nurses at Loeb have been delivering the kind of direct nursing that they believe constitutes nursing: a

philosophy of rehabilitation, direct nursing care by professional registered nurses only, and right to self-determination by the clients. (CAL)

034   NR, NAP*⁺:TM, CS

Bredenberg, V. C. *Nursing service research—experimental studies with the nursing service team.* Philadelphia: J. B. Lippincott, 1951.

Due to the changing function of the professional nurse, in response to delegation of many former functions of medicine plus movement of nursing toward professional status, nursing service has been forced to utilize nonprofessional personnel for many functions. Differentiation of nursing activities according to function or the formation of integrated nursing service teams appeared to be the only practical solutions. A functional analysis of the nursing service team indicated both quantitative and qualitative superiority to the traditional case method (Bredenberg, V. *A functional analysis of the nursing service team.* Washington, D.C.: Catholic University of America Press, 1949). This report describes further research and replication of the first study. Some conclusions were that approximately 2.0 hours per patient per day shift provided adequate care in medical-surgical units, contingent on a 1:2 proportion of professional to nonprofessional nurses. Recommendations are given on use of team plan. It is interesting to note that the comparison of case and team nursing was made on the basis of the following data: reductions of consultations with the head nurse, number of trips to the supply room and by whom, number of messenger-service trips, overtime per day by all personnel, and (in the earlier 1949 study) time spent by various personnel in giving morning care. A one-group experimental design was used, case method being the control situation and team nursing being the experimental situation. Assumptions are not all explicit. (JB)

035   NR

Brief, A. P. Turnover among hospital nurses: A suggested model. *Journal of Nursing Administration.* October 1976, 6(8):55–58.

The author considers the extent to which nurses' competency is utilized and growth challenged by their work. He suggests a model which includes lack of skill variety, task identity, autonomy, and feedback in the job, unmet expectations deriving from nursing education, and financial and social factors as variables leading to turnover. (JB)

036   NR, OS, PC, NAP⁺:TM

Brooks, E. A. Team nursing—1961. *American Journal of Nursing.* April 1961, 61: 87.

Team nursing is defined as "a means whereby the patient may receive individualized care and nursing personnel may function at their maximum potential. The Nursing Team is a group of nursing personnel working together in a team relationship to give nursing care to patients." The basic pattern for team nursing and the support systems needed, especially educational and administrative supports, are described. Staff required on each unit varies with type of patient; in general units providing complex and extensive operative procedures and medical units with a high percentage of acute coronary disease patients require more RNs and students. Units serving patients with less severe illness may be assigned a higher proportion of LPNs and aides and a lower percentage of RNs and students. (JB)

037   OS, NAP⁺:PN

Brown, B. The autonomous nurse and primary nursing. *Nursing Administration Quarterly.* Fall 1976, 1(1):31–36.

Paper adapted from presentation at the National Joint Practice Commission Program, ANA convention, 1976 in Atlantic City. Describes family-centered health care in primary nursing organizational framework. (JB)

038   OS, NAP⁺:TM

Brown, E. & Reche, J. Methods study shaped team nursing plan. *Modern Hospital.* September 1966, 107:121-3.

Team nursing was begun after a work sampling study suggested it would improve utilization of nurses. Many nonnursing tasks which had been performed by nurses were delegated to other personnel. (JB)

039   NR, OS

Brown, E. L. *Nursing reconsidered, a study of change. Part I, the professional role in institu-* *tional nursing.* Philadelphia: J. B. Lippincott Co., 1970.

This report describes new or evolving nursing roles and health programs that might provide clues or models to increase the effectiveness of nursing practice and service. Technical specialization, the expanding role of the clinical nursing specialist, and the reorganization of nursing education and nursing services in hospitals and other organizations are discussed. Current nursing practice in extended-care facilities, nursing homes, retirement homes, and homes for the aged is explored. Various models of patient care and reorganization of services, including organizational changes required to implement new "nursing roles," are described. (From *Planning for Nursing Needs and Resources,* DHEW Pub. No. (NIH) 72–87, p. 153, April 1972.)

040   PC*

Brown, J. S., Buchanan, D. & Hsu, L. Sex differences in sick role behavior during hospitalization after open heart surgery. *Research in Nursing and Health.* 1978, 1(1):37–48.

The proposition examined here is that there are sex differences in the enactment of the sick role. Specifically, in comparing the recovery of 50 male and 50 female patients following open heart surgery, it was hypothesized that male patients would (a) be transferred from the cardiac recovery room earlier, (b) be discharged from the hospital earlier, (c) achieve independence in self-care and in ambulation earlier, and (d) receive fewer pain medications and tranquilizers. Support was found only for the hypotheses of earlier hospital discharge and earlier self-care. The patient's physical condition—indicated by type of surgery, time in operating room, time on bypass, and units of blood—was related to time in recovery room and length of postoperative hospitalization. Of the variables examined, age emerged as the most powerful predictor of medication dosage, with older patients receiving significantly fewer analgesics and tranquilizers. The following conclusions were reached: (a) the salience of sex role expectations for sick role behavior varies with the particular measure considered and (b) the overall significance of sex role expectations in determining sick role behavior was slight for this sample of seriously ill patients. (Authors' abstract)

041   PC*, NR*, OS*, NAP*:CS

Brown, M. *Nurses, Patients, and Systems*. Columbia, Missouri: University of Missouri Press, 1968.

Decent and provocative study of skilled nursing care's effect on older patients, in three nursing home settings. An assumption in this study was that the older patient suffering from a chronic disease is likely to be undergoing a process of atrophy rather than development. The hypothesis was that, given certain minimum environmental conditions, this process of atrophy could be arrested and even reversed by the introduction of certain nurse-initiated interchanges of resources, designated skilled nursing care. The hypothesis was supported. Positively valued psycho-social change occurred in older persons in three controlled settings after the experimental interventions, which consisted of a specially prepared nurse caring for the same patient for one and one-half hours, 3 times a week, for 6 weeks; care included feeding and bedmaking but not medications or treatments. (JB)

042   NR, OS

Brown, R. W. Improved utilization of nurses through reorganization of the nursing division. (Unpublished master's thesis, Washington University, Dept. of Health Care Administration, 1970. Available from University Microfilm International, Ann Arbor, Mich. *Abstracts of Hospital Management Studies,* No. NU1–5842.

Theoretical presentation of schemes for optimum utilization of personnel, including consideration of skill levels, architectural design, and other variables. Based on literature review and work study analysis of data (collected by author) at Jewish Hospital. Utilization measured in terms of optimum use of nurses' time. (JB)

043   PC, NR*, NAP*:FN

Bueker, K. & Sainato, H. K. *A study of staffing patterns in psychiatric nursing.* Washington: Saint Elizabeth's Hospital, 1968.

The purpose of the study was to determine the effects of selected combinations of nursing staff with prescribed functions upon the therapeutic milieu and nursing care of patients. The results of this study showed that a selected combination of ten nursing staff, with functions prescribed by a graduate nurse, along with the services of a ward clerk and participation from the ward physician, increased the effectiveness of the ward milieu and improved the treatment program for patients. Comparison with wards that served as controls substantiated the findings reported here and elsewhere that traditional staffing patterns and only remote supervision by professional personnel, maintained status quo and custodial patient care. (Abstract from *Planning for Nursing Needs and Resources,* DHEW Pub. No. (NIH) 72–87, p. 158, April 1972.)

044   PC, NR

Carter, J. H. *Standards of nursing care: A guide for evaluation.* New York: Springer Publishing Company, 1972.

This book is a report of a two-year project focusing on: (1) the development of written standards of nursing care, (2) the development of tools for the evaluation of nursing care, and (3) the development of a technique for using the evaluation tool. The authors describe a patient classification system which was used by the Standards Committee. Three categories are described: self-care, partial care and total care. Five major areas of physical dependency upon the nursing staff were identified: (1) ambulation and movement, (2) feeding, (3) bathing, (4) elimination, and (5) activities involving special nursing intervention (monitors, therapy for hemorrhage, isolation, radiation precautions, etc.) These areas of dependency were described in terms of the three care categories. Authors describe staffing and budgeting calculations based on nursing care requirements derived from patient classification data. (JC)

045   NAP*:TM, PN

Cassata, D. M. *The effects of two patterns of nursing care on the perceptions of patients and nursing staff in two urban hospitals.* (Doctoral dissertation, University of Minnesota, 1973) Ann Arbor, Mich.: University Microfilms International, No. 74–10,492.

The major purpose of this study was primarily two-fold: (1) to examine the impact of two nursing-care systems within a state and a private hospital upon the patients' perceptions of their nursing care, and (2) to examine the impact of these two nursing-care systems on the staff's perceptions of nursing care, job satisfaction, and station effectiveness. Differences were found between primary and team nursing on a nurse affect scale, staff perceptions of care, job satisfaction, and station effectiveness. (Team nursing staff had higher job satisfaction and station effectiveness ratings). There were also significant differences between private and state hospitals on several dependent variables. Possible interaction or multivariate effects are not described. (JC)

046   OS, NAP:TM

Chi Systems, Inc. *The Friesen no-nursing station concept: Its effects on nurse staffing.* Ann Arbor, Mich.: Chi Systems, Inc., 1970.

Study objective was to determine the effect on nurse staffing of the Friesen design concepts. Changes in staffing requirements and allocation are identified. Team nursing was the assignment pattern. The Friesen design increased time spent with patients and reduced walking time and number of personnel required compared with averages in three other "conventional unit" studies. Assumptions and constraints employed to validate the comparison between this study and the other studies are described; the assignment pattern (team), charting practices, staffing patterns, and size of units were similar in all study units. Similarities and differences are described in detail only for physical, organizational, and staffing comparisons. (JB)

047   NR, NAP:PN

Christman, L. The autonomous nursing staff in the hospital. *Nursing Administration Quarterly.* Fall 1976, 1(1):37–44.

Article adapted from a presentation at the program: "Prerequisite for nurse-physician col-

laboration: Nursing autonomy," sponsored by the National Joint Practice Commission at the ANA Convention 1976. Author is Dean of the College of Nursing, Rush University, Chicago, Il. Description of organizational structure and support systems for "autonomous nursing," which includes constancy of patient assignment, 24-hour responsibility, scientifically ordered care plans, fixing of accountability, and rewards for excellence. NAP is primary nursing. Staff qualifications briefly described. (JB)

048   NAP:PN

Christman, L. NAQ forum: Primary nursing: Why not? *Nursing Administration Quarterly.* Winter 1977, 1(2):83–85.

This brief, flamboyant article describes the benefits of primary nursing in terms of quality care gains, including: (1) nurse assumes full responsibility, (2) nurse performance is measurable, (3) continuity of patient care is certain, (4) accountability for outcomes can be fixed, (5) errors of commission and omission are reduced, and (6) clinical data becomes more precise. In addition to quality care issues, primary nursing affords the following benefits: (1) more visible nursing process; (2) clearer definition of what constitutes nursing practice, (3) facilitation of practitioners becoming better role models for students, (4) self-supervision fostered, (5) enhanced opportunities for consultation, and (6) enhanced nurse-physician interdependence. (JC)

049   NAP⁺:PN

Christman, L. & Buerger, M. Primary nursing care. *Journal of Nursing Administration.* October 1976, 6(8):9.

Review by Karen L. Ciske of the dialogue between Christman and Buerger on six audio-cassette tapes (Volumes 1–6. Sawyer, Michigan: Institute of Continuing Education, 1975. $42.00). The discussion is directed primarily toward nurse administrators. Discussion covers impact on the hospital, interdisciplinary planning, research, coordination with nursing education, implementation steps, division of patient care responsibilities, and contrasts between large teaching and small community hospitals. (JB)

050 NR, OS, NAP:FN

Christman, L. P. & Jelinek, R. C. Old patterns waste half the nursing hours. *Modern Hospital.* January 1967, 108(1):78–81.

These authors report that the organizational arrangement of the process of care determines the use of all types of personnel. Because of the scarce supply of trained manpower, the form of the organization is particularly important when considering the effective use of professional personnel. They contend that nursing care can be of no greater quality than the training of the person giving the direct care. In addressing the problems inherent in "functional" nursing, the authors cite the following: (1) Care of patients is fragmented. (2) Unassigned tasks frequently are not done. (3) Status becomes attached to the amounts of undesirable and low-level tasks one is assigned. (4) Salaries become attached to role positions rather than to competence with patients. (5) The training of RNs is wasted. (6) Patients are deprived of anywhere from 50–75 percent of RN care. Recommended solutions include: (1) service-unit supervisor who deals mainly with nonclinical activities, (2) utility aides–a person who performs lower-level tasks and would be assigned to the same RN and the same patients everyday, (3) unit-chief nurse who functions as person with "clinical" authority, and (4) use of clinical nursing specialists to assist staff nurses to take on clinical roles. (JC)

051 NR*, OS*, NAP*:FN

Christman, N. J. Clinical performance of baccalaureate graduates. *Nursing Outlook.* January 1971, 19(1):54–56.

This article reports an analysis of the nursing care given by baccalaureate degree graduates in four practice settings that used different methods of patient care assignment. Two agencies using functional method and two agencies using unit management were studied. No random selection was done; the Slater nursing competencies rating scale was the evaluation tool. Findings were: No association was found between level of performance and length of employment in either type of structure, or year of graduation. The most recent graduates in functional setting had lower scores than those in unit management setting. The mean Slater scores for graduates on unit management set-tings were significantly higher than mean Slater scores for graduates on functional units. (T=significant at the 0.05 level). Additional findings: The areas of teaching, rehabilitation, and involvement of the patient in care yielded lower scores in both patient care assignment settings. The subjects in unit management, however, were able to maintain a higher level of performance in these three areas. (JC)

052 NR, OS, NAP⁺:PN

Cicatiello, J. NAQ forum: Primary nursing: Why not? *Nursing Administration Quarterly.* Winter 1977, 1(2):82–83.

This brief article describes the positive results and problems encountered in implementing primary nursing. Positive results include: (1) increased continuity of care, (2) less fragmentation of patient care, (3) greater personal rapport between nurse and patient, (4) increased trust of patient in the nurse, (5) faster patient recuperation, (6) more job satisfaction for the nurse, (7) improved interpersonal relations with all allied health disciplines, and (8) improved patient teaching. Problems encountered in implementing primary nursing include: (1) nurses and allied health disciplines have not always understood the role of the primary nurse, (2) turnover of nursing personnel presents many problems, (3) language barriers between patient and nurse can be a communication problem, (4) staff, at times, revert back to team nursing, (5) shift rotation leads to changes in primary nurse assignment, and (6) not all physicians were supportive of the concept. (JC)

053 NR, OS, NAP⁺:PN

Ciske, K. L. Primary nursing: An organization that promotes professional practice. *Journal of Nursing Administration.* January-February 1974, 4(1):28–31.

Overview (18 mos. later) of process through which changes in the organization and delivery of nursing care on a 23-bed medical unit were accomplished. Hospital nursing has been a difficult place to implement professional practice. In an attempt to find ways to improve the delivery of nursing care and the level of staff satisfaction, a group of nurses at the University of Minnesota Hospitals adapted the one-to-one assignment model to a small patient unit. Decision making was decentralized to the nurse who knew the patient best, the primary nurse. Because of his or her role in staff development, the head nurse was seen to be pivotal to the success of primary nursing. The author is developing an independent nursing role as a consultant/instructor/ facilitator for primary nursing. (CAL)

054   NR, NAP*:PN, TM

Ciske, K. L. Primary nursing evaluation. *American Journal of Nursing.* 1974, 74(8):1436–1438.

Subjective and objective responses briefly presented describe staff and patient satisfaction with primary nursing in an attempt to answer the question, "Does primary nursing facilitate what nursing has to offer?" The author, a clinician who worked with the initial primary nursing unit and in the primary nursing study group at the University of Minnesota, describes indexes of effectiveness and acceptance of primary nursing, including the shortcomings of a patient questionnaire she helped to construct. Findings show lower turnover among RNs and LPNs on primary unit. (CAL)

055   NR, NAP⁺:PN

Ciske, K. L. Misconceptions about staffing and patient assignment in primary nursing. *Nursing Administration Quarterly.* Winter 1977, 1(2): 61–68.

This consultant identifies two major areas of confusion regarding the practical application of primary nursing: staffing and patient assignment. In addressing the issue of staffing, the author discusses utilization of LPNs, aides, part-time RNs, and the head nurse's role. In addressing the problem of patient assignment, the author cites the following "principles:" (1) equal case load, depending on staff ability and hours, (2) optimum match between patient need and staff competence, (3) a variety of patient conditions for staff growth, and (4) the geographical location of rooms. In terms of duration of assignment, many misconceptions about primary nursing have emerged. For very long-term patients where nurses and clients experience personality clashes, assignments are changed. When a patient is readmitted, the choice to remain the primary nurse is left to the nurse. (JC)

056   PC

Clark, E. L. & Diggs, W. W. Quantifying patient care needs. *Hospitals.* September 16, 1971, 45:96.

The authors evaluate the PETO method for assessing patient care needs. The method was implemented with the hope that it would be a more accurate index of patient care needs than those presently available, such as census, patient days, beds, nursing hours per patient day, nursing hours per bed, per diem cost. The PETO method is for quantifying physical needs only. Authors determined that implementation of the PETO method on a pediatric unit for one year resulted in administrators being able to obtain more accurate cost figures and a more balanced budget, a decrease in nursing staff turnover, and improved staffing. The PETO method also helped explain why children's hospitals operate at a higher cost than short-term general hospitals. An infant typically consumes 20 points of care and a toddler 12 points, in contrast to an adult's 4 points, before medical orders are written. (JC)

057   PC

Cochran, J. & Derr, D. Patient acuity system for nurse staffing. *Hospital Progress.* 1975. 56(11): 51–54.

The study discusses the development and implementation of nurse staffing standards based on the time required to care for various types of patients, i.e., patient acuity categories. A staffing model was developed for each nursing unit using these standards and the mix of patients and census; the "true" variability in staffing requirements could then be determined, and better staffing patterns and mechanisms could be developed. The staffing mechanism employed was to be dynamic: it would project both census and acuity mix of patients sufficiently, prior to shift change, to properly and objectively allocate staff resources. The article presents acuity definitions for rehabilitation. Team nursing was utilized on this unit. (JPK)

058   NAP*:PN, TM

Collins, V. B. *The primary nursing role as a model for evaluating quality of patient care, patient satisfaction, job satisfaction, and cost effectiveness in an acute care setting.* (Doctoral dissertation, University of Utah, 1975) Ann Arbor, Mich.: University Microfilms International, No. 75-22, 117.

This study of primary nursing is based on the premise that a unique organizational structure in an acute care setting will (1) improve quality levels of nursing care, (2) maximize cost effectiveness, and (3) increase job satisfaction and promote patient satisfaction. The Nursing Service Department of two general acute care hospitals provided the clinical laboratory for data collection. The instrument developed for evaluating quality of care included items from nationally accepted instruments for measuring quality of nursing care. The items most nearly representative of the primary care philosophy were abstracted. The sample population for quality care included 480 audits containing 30 variables for a total of 14,400 responses. An experimental (primary nursing) versus a control (team nursing) unit formed the basis for this research design. From the primary nursing unit there was significant evidence that early and more meaningful assessment of patient needs resulted. The patient progress reports indicated the therapeutic nursing interventions resulted in planning care to meet the patient's needs. The data further concluded that continuity of care and discharge planning for follow-up was positively endorsed, and the patient identification of his nurse was meaningful. During the three-month period, the following additional data were collected: (1) cost analysis relative to the individual unit staff component; (2) job satisfaction inventory utilizing a job satisfaction questionnaire that had proven high validity and reliability—a pre and posttest design was introduced with a total of 83 questionnaires completed; and (3) a total of 191 patient satisfaction post-discharge telephone interviews were conducted for all available patients released from the experimental and control units. The data from the quality of care results were analyzed by applying the chi square test for probability of difference. The items of significance were focused on the following topics: (1) assessment of the patient family needs as initial preparation for care, (2) maintenance of a current written nursing care plan for each patient based on patient/family physical, emotional, and teaching needs, (3) improvement of discharge planning and home care, and (4) documentation of collaborative efforts between disciplines and assessment of patient progress. The findings conclude that primary nursing as an organizational modality significantly improved the quality of patient care, over team nursing. The cost factors were negligible in impact, indicating that variations in salary compensation make it difficult to compute consistent data. The null hypothesis of no difference was not rejected. In the Job Satisfaction Inventory an attempt was made to identify the specific primary nurse with the patient's satisfaction. This resulted in a small sample. Even though there was significant difference in one hospital, the total analysis of the dependent t test resulted in rejection of the hypothesis. The patient satisfaction sample was computed with a chi square test for probability of difference. There was a high significance in the data from the primary nurse unit exposing the patient's willingness to return to the hospital. It was felt that this was good indication that the patient was better satisfied and would be more willing to return to that unit, if necessary. (Author's abstract)

059   NAP*

Comstock, D. W. & Scott, W. R. Technology and the structure of subunits: Distinguishing individual and workgroup effects. *Administration Science Quarterly,* June 1977, 22(2):177-202.

This paper develops and tests the argument that technology should be thought of as representing the work of each level of organization as well as different subunits in an organization. Predictions of divergent effects of individual task and subunit workflow technologies on staff characteristics and subunit structures were tested on 142 patient care wards in a stratified random sample of 16 hospitals. The data clearly support the conclusion that as we move from tasks to workflow, the effects of technological predictability shift from individual job qualifications and specialization to systems of subunit coordination and control. The effects of technology are compared to those of subunit size, and it is concluded that while size continues to have independent effects, it is a less powerful predictor of subunit structure than technology. (Authors' abstract)

060   OS*

Condon, T. B. A. A unit management evaluation. *Hospitals.* November 16, 1974, 48:61-62.

This article is an evaluative report of the unit management system at Yale-New Haven Hospital that freed nurses from nonnursing functions and thereby allowed them to redirect their time into the performance of patient-centered activities. A distinct unit management department was established that reported directly to hospital administration. (This was not within the nursing department.) This department was charged with five major responsibilities usually performed by the head nurse: (1) service coordination, (2) patient assistance, (3) maintenance of supply and equipment, (4) secretarial management, and (5) budget monitoring. Unfortunately, the methodology used to evaluate this system is poorly reported. Findings were: (1) staff on experimental unit perceived an increased proefficiency in floor performance, and (2) staff on experimental unit perceived an improvement in morale and job satisfaction. (JC)

061   PC

Connor, R. J. *A hospital inpatient classification system.* (Doctoral dissertation, Johns Hopkins University, Baltimore, Maryland, 1960) Ann Arbor, Mich.: University Microfilms International, No. 60-3,319.

(This early study of nurse activities is referred to by many later works.) This dissertation presents a hospital inpatient classification system which relates the time spent by nursing personnel with a patient to his classification. The implications of such a system to hospitals are discussed. A work sampling study which recognized the variations in nursing patient care loads and led to the development of theoretical models for the total nursing work load on a ward is presented. Alternative hospital staffing systems are discussed in light of these results. Analytical and simulated comparisons of the present staffing system and a controlled variable staffing system are presented. The results of the comparisons indicate a controlled variable staffing system permits better utilization of personnel as well as a reduction in personnel. (Author's abstract)

062   NR, PC

Connor, R. J. A work sampling study of variations in nursing workload. *Hospitals.* May 1, 1961, 35: 40.

This article reports on a work sampling study conducted to investigate causes for variations in the direct care index. Among the findings, the author reports that as nursing hours available increase, there is no increase in direct patient care but, instead, an increase in personal time. Further analysis of time in direct patient care indicated that it is not significantly related to the nursing personnel hours available. Analysis of time in productive activity showed that total work load does vary significantly with the direct care index and with hours available, but not with census. (JC)

063   PC

Connor, R. J., Flagle, C. D., Preston, R. & Singer, S. Effective use of nursing resources: A research report. *Hospitals.* May 1, 1961, 35:30–39.

A system of patient classification by severity of illness to determine nursing requirements on a day-to-day basis is described by the authors in this research report. How demands for certain supplies, such as linen, can also be predicted through this system is also explained. Through time studies on direct patient care activities of the nursing staff, 3 levels of patient classifications were derived: I = Self care, II = Partial care, III = Total care. These categories were based on the following patient areas: (1) mobility, (2) emotional state, (3) level of consciousness, (4) adequacy of vision, and (5) need for isolation. By utilizing this classification system, a total direct care index per unit per day can be determined and used by administrators in staffing decisions. (JC)

064   OS*, NAP:TM

Cope, M. J. *The effect of unit reorganization on nursing personnel utilization and patient welfare.* (Unpublished doctoral dissertation, University of Utah, Department of Educational Administration, August 1967.)

The study ascertains the effects on: (1) certain levels of hospital activities (administration, nursing, clerical, housekeeping, dietary, messenger, and unclassified); (2) certain areas of hospital activities (patient-centered, personnel-centered, unit-centered and other-centered), and (3) certain patient welfare ratings (mental attitude, mobility, and physical independence); when a nursing unit was reorganized from a traditional structure using a head nurse to one which incorporated the use of a clinical nurse specialist and a ward management system. Team nursing remained the nursing assignment pattern. (JB)

065   OS, NR, NAP⁺*:PN

Corn, F., Hahn, M. & Lepper, K. Salvaging primary nursing. *Supervisor Nurse.* May 1977, 8(5):19–21, 24–25.

This is a description of an unsuccessful demonstration project intended to provide comprehensive patient care on a surgical unit at Bronx Municipal Hospital Center. The project died prematurely, a victim of staff shortages resulting from New York City's fiscal crisis. The time and effort of six months was expended by staff in the preparation and implementation of the primary nursing care project. Despite the early termination, the nursing staff accepted the concept of primary nursing care and continues to implement it on a limited basis. This article presents the problems and outcomes of the project. (CAL)

066   NAP⁺:TM, PN

Corpuz, T. Primary nursing meets needs, expectations of patients and staff. *Hospitals.* June 1, 1977, 51:95–100.

This article describes how a task force of industrial engineers, management consultants and a clinical nursing specialist evaluated nursing care delivery under the "team nursing" system. They found that nurse aides were not being effectively utilized—as much as 60 percent of their time was not related to patient needs and that RN team leaders spent most of their time administering medications. The task force concluded that the patient was receiving the least amount of care from the person most prepared to provide that care. "Modular" nursing was developed as an alternate system for the delivery of nursing care. The remainder of the article describes implementation and the positive evaluation of primary nursing; equivalent cost (to team nursing), improved quality of process, greater job satisfaction, greater continuity and improved learning for patients are reported. (JC)

067   NR*

Corwin, R. G. The professional employee: A study of conflict in nursing roles. In Skipper, J. K. & Leonard, R. C. (eds.) *Social Interaction and Patient Care,* pp. 341–356. Philadelphia: J. B. Lippincott Company, 1965.

A study of the effect of educational preparation on role conflicts and discrepancy after graduation; degree and diploma students and graduates are compared on role conceptions. Hypothesis was that after graduation, convergence of professional and bureaucratic principles would produce conflict in roles, and that graduates of degree programs would be more vulnerable to such conflict because of the independence of the nursing program from hospital administration. The hypothesis was generally supported. The author concludes that individuals adjust to the conflicts imposed by the structure of their work but the result may be compromise in the performance of roles. (JB)

068   OS⁺, NAP⁺:PN, TM

Cox, B., Anderson, J. & Page, J. The expanded role of the nurse: A systems analysis. *Nursing Papers.* Spring 1976, 8:26–44.

Focusing on decision making and the problem-solving process, the investigators examined three psychiatric units which have primary nursing care, team nursing, and primary nurse therapists. Many assessment tools were employed, including researcher observation, a 30-item agree/disagree questionnaire on nursing practice on the particular ward, an 8-hour diary of actual nursing activity, and a sociogram illustrating staff interactions. Findings indicated that only 50 percent of nursing time was spent in direct care, the rest being primarily involved in staff meetings. Nurses apparently suffered from "communication overload." Communication activities were not valued by the nurses. The primary care unit had the most direct communication patterns and the highest job satisfaction. It appeared that nurses had assumed the primary therapist role as a consequence of decreased numbers of medical staff. While the nurses were pleased with their new responsibilities and knowledge, they had difficulty finding sufficient time and being formally recognized and accepted by other staff; they felt they needed more training and supervision.

There was much independent decision making, usually involving overall assessment of individual patients, planning of daily patient care, and work management. Independent decision-making behavior decreased when other health professionals were present. In group situations nurses were less assertive and deferred decision making to others. The study documents a trend toward more responsibility by nurses; the extended role is becoming well established. (Abstract from *Nursing Research,* Jan.–Feb., 1977, 26(1):72)

069   PC, NAP*:PN, TM

Daeffler, R. J. Patients' perception of care under team and primary nursing. *Journal of Nursing Administration.* March-April 1975, 20–26.

This article deals with the tension-reducing effects of expressive nursing activities and with primary nursing as an assignment system that allows more room for these activities than team nursing. A study of perceptions of care in 82 hospitalized patients showed higher satisfaction and less omissions in care reported by patients in a primary care unit than in team nursing units. (JB)

070   OS⁺

Davis, B. C., Bealcher, J., Felming, M. & McCormack, M. Implementation of problem oriented charting in a large, regional community hospital. *Journal of Nursing Administration.* Nov.-Dec. 1974, 4(6):33–41.

The problem oriented system of charting (POSC) was instituted at the Western Pennsylvania Hospital after a one-year program of study, planning, and teaching. The adoption of POSC has brought improvements not only in charting and data processing, but also in the level of the relationships between members of the health team and the patients. (JB)

071   NR*

Davis, B. G. Effect of levels of nursing education on patient care: A replication. *Nursing Research.* March-April 1974, 23(2):150–155.

The purpose of this study was: (1) to assess differences in skill possessed by the clinical nurse specialist, the BSN, and the diploma nurse (the effect of education on performance), (2) to assess the effect of increased or greater number of years of, clinical experience on the quality and quantity of nursing care, and (3) to assess the effect of area specialization on the quality and quantity of nursing care. Results are: (1) Clinical nurse specialists made significantly more relevant observations, suggested a greater number of relevant actions and gave more appropriate reasons for the actions taken than BSN or diploma nurses. (2) Increased experience depressed rather than enhanced quality of performance. Even an advanced degree was not sufficient to alter the negative effects of extended experience on performance. (3) When transference of nursing skills from one specialty to other areas of nursing was analyzed for 50 med-surg nurses and 37 psychiatric nurses, no significant differences were found. (JC)

072   OS

del Bueno, D. Organizing and staffing the in-service department. *Journal of Nursing Administration.* December 1976, 6(10):12–13.

Discussion of what kinds of people and what in-service organizational structure best promote employee competence. Stress is given to the working philosophy and relationships of the people in the organization. Qualifications of the director of the in-service department are discussed. (JB)

073   OS, NR, NAP⁺:TM

Deming, E. A. A practicing system for professional nursing. *Nursing Clinics of North America.* June 1971, 6(6):311–320.

Description of an organizational pattern for nursing care in a general hospital, based on identification of values fundamental to the nursing process and facilitation of a climate that would suport these values when implemented. The nursing assignment pattern was team nursing, with a professional nurse administering an integral part of the patient's care. A head nurse and assistant head nurse provided leadership for the nursing care program of a designated group of patients (average number=27) over a 24-hour period. Patients' care plans and profiles were revised throughout their stay. Effectiveness of care was evaluated by the team and nurse clinician. Patient care was not confined to the hospital setting but a system of communication was maintained with other patient-care disciplines and community agencies. Nurse clinicians were introduced after the program of team nursing was established. Interdisciplinary communication and use of specialists, including psychiatric nurses, are part of the structure. (BK)

074   OS, NAP⁺:TM

Denn, N. Where can nurses practice as they're taught? *American Journal of Nursing.* December 1974, 74(12):2212–2215.

Description of the attempted implementation and failure of a proposal by seven new graduate nurses to change practices on an acute medical pediatric unit. The author reports that failure was due to lack of support and implementation by nursing administration. The proposal included 24-hour coverage by RNs, team nursing, and interdisciplinary and staff communication structures. The previous assignment pattern is not described. (BK)

075   NAP*:PN, TM

Dewey, C. Comparison of quality of care in two pediatric patient care systems: Team versus primary care nursing. (Unpublished master's thesis, The University of Rochester, 1974.) Available from University Microfilms International, Ann Arbor, Mich. *Abstracts of Hospital Management Studies,* No. 15016 NU.

The purpose of this research was to examine the effect of two forms of nursing organization, team nursing and primary care nursing, on the quality of patient care. A static group comparative design was used to generate testable hypotheses for larger and more controlled studies. The Munley instrument, which objectively measures the quality of patient care, was adapted by the researcher to include tasks specific to pediatric patient care. The adopted instrument examined observable nurse-client interaction, patient care plans, charted notes, and responses from interviews with parents. One pediatric unit was used to examine both systems of organization. The setting was observed by the researcher while team nursing was practiced and again six months later under primary care nursing. During each period of investigation random assignment of 20 patients to the study

was determined by a toss of a coin. Each patient was then blocked into a medical or surgical category. Data were analyzed in percentages of difference between and among groups on overall needs and separately for each of the nine categories of needs. Overall analysis of the data indicated an advantage of primary care nursing in all but two categories: (1) spiritual needs and (2) medications. In no category did team nursing establish a higher percentage of favorable responses. The greatest difference occurred within the expressive and communication categories. There were more RNs staffing the unit during primary nursing phase. (JC)

076   OS

Dickman, R. Relationship of communication to job satisfaction: Nursing as a special case. (Unpublished master's thesis, University of Washington, School of Nursing, 1974.)

The purpose of this study was to test the hypothesis that nurses' perception of communication within a hospital complex co-varies positively with job satisfaction. The problem was whether lack of communication created job dissatisfaction due to poor personal attitudes, tension, less coordination between departments, and less role clarity between the nurses themselves. The data were obtained from a questionnaire distributed to staff nurses employed in two general hospitals of 200 beds. A total of 60 questionnaires were distributed and 49 responded. The data indicated that job satisfaction was related to communication and the lack of communication could affect the productivity of the staff nurses. The approach or attitude of the communicator can affect the receiver. Tension appeared to be a prime factor relating to communication. Tension can create conflict and cause the nurses to develop false perceptions from lack of listening. The nurses look for clues in communication that only support their own arguments. Also, there was a lack of upward flow of communication. Their opinions were sought but not often used. The nurses need to have role clarification to become more productive. Lack of role clarification and administrative support can lead to lack of cooperation among the nurses themselves or between other hospital-related groups. The staff nurses need interaction among their own group and other hospital groups to foster participation in hospital activities and develop a sense of belonging to their own group and to the hospital. (Abstracted in Western Interstate Commission for Higher Education in Nursing, *Newly Initiated and Completed Research,* Vol. 11, December 1975.)

077   NR*

DiMarco, N., Carter, J. H., Castels, M. R. & Corrigan, M. K. Nursing resources on the nursing unit and quality of patient care. *International Journal of Nursing Studies.* 1976, 13(3): 139–152.

This article deals with the relationships between nursing resources and quality of patient care. The following relationships were found: (1) The quality of the nursing care plan was negatively related to the number of part-time student nurses, full-time aides, part-time RNs, and full-time RNs. (2) The quality of the nursing record was negatively related to the number of part-time RNs and full-time student nurses. (3) The quality of the nursing care at the bedside was negatively related to the number of full-time student nurses and number of patients on the ward. (4) The total quality of nursing care was negatively related to the number of full-time student nurses, part-time RNs, part-time student nurses, full-time aides, and full-time RNs. The results are discussed in terms of the effects various nursing resources have on the performance of the RN. (CAL)

078   OS*, NAP*:TM

Dornblaser, B. M. & Piedmont, E. B. *Spoke design for inpatient care—final report.* National Center for Health Services Research and Development, DHEW, 1969.

This study is concerned with three problems: (1) to improve patient welfare within the amount of registered nurse time available and expended, for inpatient care, (2) to reduce the amount of capital funds required for inpatient care facilities, both in the short and long run, and (3) to reduce the rate of increase in the expense of operating the inpatient facility. The study focuses on physical and organizational changes directed toward these three objectives. There were six study units in all; four were identified as having team nursing; the other two NAPs are not specified. The teams consisted of one RN, one LPN, and one aide. The head nurse position was eliminated and the duties of that position

reallocated to the supervisor, clinical nurse specialist, and support personnel. Environmental changes were made to facilitate keeping nursing personnel at the bedside. Work satisfaction increased slightly for the entire nursing staff in the experimental design units; in some instances, work satisfaction was related to workload and other variables. Turnover rates and patient satisfaction and welfare scores were unchanged. The elimination of the head nurse position was largely successful. Tasks performed by the head nurses were allocated to the small nursing teams and to other administrative positions. (JC)

079   NAP

Douglass, L. M. *Review of team nursing.* St. Louis: C. V. Mosby Co., 1973.

General review of team nursing and the historical background of nursing, with particular emphasis on the emergence of the nurse leader. Other topics covered include a theoretical basis for the study of nursing action, review of the problem-solving approach, nurse characteristics and climates that influence behavior, processes involved in delegation of authority, group dynamics and communication, and planning for evaluation of the nursing process. Author views team nursing as "the answer" to helping nurses cope with the multiplicity of responsibilities they now have. Case, functional, and other modes of delivering nursing care are also defined. (JB)

080, 081   NAP:TM

Douglass, L. & Bevis, E. *Nursing leadership in action.* 2nd edition. St. Louis: C. V. Mosby, 1974.

This book is an attempt to elaborate a theoretical framework for staff nursing that will enable the nurse to mobilize all available resources for the benefit of patients. Other goals are to provide a body of knowledge that will supply a theoretical framework of administrative principles for use by the nurse-leader, to provide a practical method for utilization of these administrative principles in day-to-day nursing activities, and to promote a habit of mind in the nurse practitioner that will transform the nurse utilizing these methods into an effective leader. These objectives are met through a consideration of the staff nurse as a team leader and the formulation and utilization of principles necessary for effective team functioning. A third edition of this book has been published. (Adapted from preface)

082   OS, NAP:TM

Downs, R. F. Nursing in a Friesen hospital. *Supervisor Nurse.* March 1971, 39–43.

This article discusses the methods and resources necessary to implement a Friesen hospital. According to the author, a Friesen-planned hospital incorporates a "total system" of nursing and patient care and is supported by four major characteristics: (1) no nursing station, (2) a supply system which brings materials directly to the nurse, (3) a reorganization of nursing that relieves nurses of all paranursing functions, and (4) a communications system which provides instantaneous message sending and receiving capabilities. Team nursing is identified as a fundamental requirement to the successful implementation of the Friesen nursing and patient care concept. (JC)

083   PC*, NAP*

Dumas, R. G., Anderson, B. J. & Leonard, R. C. The importance of the expressive function in preoperative preparation. In Skipper, J. K. and Leonard, R. C. *Social Interaction and Patient Care, pp. 16–29.* Philadelphia: J. B. Lippincott Company, 1965.

Report of the effects of psychological preparation of surgical patients by a nurse, on the incidence of postoperative vomiting and implications for including expressive care functions in the patient care equation. A single nurse assessed, planned, intervened, and evaluated the care. The nurse was prepared at the graduate level. (JB)

084   PC, NR, OS, NAP⁺:PN

Eagen, Sister M. C. New staffing pattern allows for total individual quality care. *Hospital Progress.* February 1970, 51(2):62–64.

The author defines "total individual quality care" as "the assessment and planned care of each individual patient by a registered nurse." The registered nurse attempts to meet the needs of the patient either through her own profes-

sional capabilities or with the assistance of specialists in various disciplines. Functional care and team nursing care are both considered to be "traditional care" by the author. The pilot unit was staffed by registered nurses, nursing assistants, and a ward clerk on the morning and afternoon shifts. Only registered nurses were employed on the night shift. All direct patient care was provided by the registered nurses. The nursing assistants and ward clerks were under the direct supervision of the registered nurses. Nursing assistants helped the nurse in all areas not directly associated with patient care. The ward clerk acted as a receptionist and performed selected clerical work, including the copying of physicians' orders, within the nursing unit. To avoid fragmented, depersonalized care, each registered nurse was responsible for total individual quality care for five or six patients on the unit. This article describes the planning for the new staffing pattern, the in-service education required, the revision of job descriptions, and the plans for transferring and placing personnel (e.g., the head nurse, the licensed practical nurse, and the nursing aide positions were eliminated). (From *Planning for Nursing Needs and Resources,* DHEW Pub. No. (NIH) 72–87, p. 161, April 1972.)

085   NAP

Ellis, B. Nursing profession undergoes intensive scrutiny and adjustment. *Hospitals.* April 1, 1977, 51(7):139–144.

Review of the 1976 nursing literature and comments on role ambiguity, staffing, innovations in structure, autonomous nursing, and nurses as change agents in the health system. Good review and bibliography. (JB)

086   PC, OS⁺, NAP⁺:PN

Elpern, E. H. Structural and organizational supports for primary nursing. *Nursing Clinics of North America.* June 1977, 12(2):205–219.

The author was formerly unit leader on the unit described in this paper. She presents a report of the transition from team-functional to primary-modular nursing. Although not analytical or scientific in approach, this article does identify important variables—organizational and nursing resources—that were considered while implementing primary nursing. One of the more significant statements made by the author is, "There is growing recognition and appreciation that contextual variables, i.e., those that relate to the organization or environment in which care is given, are important determinants of both the process and outcomes of nursing care" (p. 205). (CAL)

087   NAP:TM

Esposito, P. & Lobozzo, S. *A manual for team nursing.* St. Louis: The Catholic Hospital Association, 1968.

A manual explaining the principles and implementation of team nursing. The roles, responsibilities, and relationship of the members of the professional health team, and particularly of the nursing team segment, are outlined. Assignment planning, team conferences, and nursing care plans are explained. Criteria for team reports are given, as are specimens of report and assignment forms and an example of a nursing team conference. (From *Abstracts of Hospital Management Studies.* June 1970, 4:141)

088   OS*

Everly, G. S. & Falcione, R. L. Perceived dimensions of job satisfaction for staff registered nurses. *Nursing Research.* September-October 1976, 25(5):346–348.

To measure the importance of dimensions of job satisfaction, 144 female registered staff nurses in four east-coast metropolitan hospitals were given an 18-item, Likert-type instrument. Results indicated that the traditional intrinsic/extrinsic dichotomy, which exists in elements of job satisfaction, did not apply. The nurses perceived their job satisfaction in a more complex fashion, in that four statistically independent dimensions emerged. They were: (1) relationship orientation, (2) internal work rewards, (3) external work rewards, and (4) administrative policies. The first factor accounted for almost 24 percent of the total variance and was the most frequently occurring factor. The study implies that previous considerations in job satisfaction for the professional may need to be reexamined in terms beyond the traditional intrinsic/extrinsic dichotomy. Other findings: Good relationship orientation, high internal work rewards, high external work rewards, and high administrative policies increased registered nurse job satisfaction. (JPK)

089   NR

Fagin, C. M. The clinical specialist as supervisor. *Nursing Outlook.* January 1967, 15(1): 34–36.

This article suggests that clinical specialists are supervisors in that they help practitioners develop clinical skills via the following: (1) functioning as role models, (2) being participant-observers involved in patient care, (3) teaching formally and informally, (4) instigating new ideas, and (5) evaluating staff performance. (JC)

090   NR*, NAP*:PN, TM

Felton, G. Increasing the quality of nursing care by introducing the concept of primary care nursing: A model project. *Nursing Research.* January-February 1975, 24(1):27–32.

This study evaluates selected variables related to quality of nursing care and cost effectiveness as they are affected by primary and group nursing assignment patterns. Nurses on an experimental unit were trained to use primary care, that is, assignment of six to eight patients to one nurse who was responsible for the planning, implementation, evaluation, and coordination of the nursing care until the patients' discharge. On a control unit, nurses participated in delivery of group care, so that the care of each patient was assigned to various nurses. Performance of the nursing care was measured by the Slater Nursing Competencies scale, the Quality Patient Care scale, and the Phaneuf Nursing Audit. Mean scores on the three instruments were found to be higher on the experimental unit. Although total hours of professional care were greater in the experimental unit, the control unit gave a larger number of hours of care (professional and nonprofessional) per patient per day; patient census accounted for the difference. Cost per patient per day was $30.14 in the experimental unit, $34.49 in the control unit. The level of educational preparation of staff was higher on the experimental unit. (Author's abstract adapted)

091   OS⁺,NAP:TM

Fielding, V. V. New team plan frees nurses to nurse. *Modern Hospital.* May 1967, 108(5):122–124.

This article summarizes the implementation of a "unified nursing plan." Whatever type of NAP existed prior to this plan is not specified. The author indicates that there are some surface similarities between the unified nursing plan and the ward management system but points out one fundamental difference, "The ward management system involves dual authority between manager and head nurse while our system gives total authority to the head nurse." The remainder of the article goes on to describe the realignment of duties to team leaders, team members, etc. The plan made possible a decrease in both the size of the nursing staff and the proportion of RNs required, resulting in cost savings. (JC)

092   PC⁺, NR

Fine, R. B. Controlling nurses workloads. *American Journal of Nursing*. December 1974, 74(12): 2206–2207.

Controlling the number of patients admitted to a rehabilitation unit who were classified as Class III (most severe) lead to more effective care and a satisfying workload for the nurses. The controlled workload is also reported to have led to increased organization, increased teamwork, increased quality of care, increased teaching of patient and family, increased patient independence, and total patient care. (BK)

093   NR

Flint, R. T. & Spensley, K. C. Recent issues in nursing manpower: A review. *Nursing Research*. May-June 1968, 18(3):217–229.

The summary of a literature review was done by two individuals with academic preparation in educational counseling. The topics reviewed include: summaries and projections for manpower, analytical studies of staffing, sociological/psychological studies of nursing students, nursing education, recruitment, supportive personnel, innovations such as tape recorders for reports, and attrition and turnover rates among nursing personnel. The authors' discussion includes the following points: (1) It is no longer necessary to specify the extent of nursing personnel shortage. Suggestions are needed as to how to affect it significantly. (2) Studies done on the sociological/psychological characteristics

of nursing students are poorly controlled and use unreliable instruments. The authors suggest that several sources of personnel have been neglected including men, the poor, and the older person. (3) The most significant reduction of personnel shortages have resulted from systematic analyses of staffing patterns, personnel utilization, and cost-benefit ratios. (4) The professional-technical categorization of nurses is not the most functional way of classifying nursing personnel. Detailed analyses of and prescriptions for the roles of the various categories of nurses is called for, including a review of the areas in which they overlap. (JC)

094   NAP:TM

Fogt, J. Team nursing: Concept and procedures. *Hospital Progress*. February 1964, 45(1):65–67.

This article reviews the evolution of team nursing after World War II and those factors which provided impetus to team nursing. The author emphasizes that team nursing is not meant to be a panacea for the nursing shortage. It is not a method for accomplishing a large amount of work with an inadequate staff. But rather, it is a system which attempts to encourage personnel to function to the limit of their potential. Advantages of team nursing are cited: (1) Lesser trained personnel are continuously supervised. Team nursing, with its decentralization, involves not only the head nurse but also the team leader in supervision. The author contends that improved patient care is a result of more closely supervised workers. (2) Team nursing provides comprehensive, individualized, and continuous care since the number of people caring for any patient is limited. (3) The professional nurse's judgement skills are available to a larger number of patients. (JC)

095   NR*

Forest, B. L. *The utilization of associate degree nursing graduates in general hospitals*. (Doctoral dissertation, Columbia University, 1965) Ann Arbor, Mich.: University Microfilms International, No. 65–14967.

Study of whether associate degree nursing graduates employed in general hospitals in New York City were performing the functions for which they had been prepared in their educational programs. The functions of a nursing team member are described as giving general nursing care with supervision and assisting in planning and evaluation of care. The majority of the AD graduates were performing functions for which they had been prepared. 80 percent were in staff nurse positions; over 90 percent of these spent more than one half of their time in performing the technical functions of nursing. The majority of the graduates also reported performing additional activities other than those for which they had received basic preparation. These included clerical, managerial role, cleaning, and medical-technical activities. AD graduates were considered for promotion on the same basis as other nurses. In making the decision to promote to head nurse, little or no consideration was given by nursing service administrators to the objectives of educational programs or the preservice preparation of the graduates of these programs. The majority of the graduates said they were not prepared to be team leaders, be in charge of the unit, or to oversee the work of others, but some did perform these duties. In some instances, in-service training prepared them for these duties; practically all AD graduates promoted to head nurse positions were trained through in-service education of some kind, had gained experience in nursing before promotion, and were promoted primarily on the basis of "ability." (JB)

096   PC*

Fortin, F. & Kirouac, S. A randomized controlled trial of pre-operative patient education. *International Journal of Nursing Studies.* 1976, 13:11–24.

The purpose of this study was to evaluate the efficacy and efficiency of a nursing intervention (pre-op teaching) in the management of selected and representative elective surgical patients. Evidence was focused on the appropriateness of instituting an ongoing structured pre-operative educational program for elective surgical patients. Education was included as part of already established preadmission procedures. A subordinate objective of the study was to develop, adapt, and validate data-gathering instruments suitable for the evaluation of patients' physical functional capacity. Technical and education aspects of care are briefly described. (CAL)

097   PC

Fralic, M. F. Developing a viable patient education program—a nursing director's perspective. *Journal of Nursing Administration.* September 1976, 6(7):30–36.

Recognizing professional and moral obligations for educational intervention, Braddock General Hospital created a viable, meaningful teaching program. It responds to patient needs, is professionally satisfying to the staff, and is a notably cost-effective effort. Specific teaching protocols are presented for diabetic, ostomy and MI patients. The nursing assignment pattern is not described. Responsibility for teaching was given to staff nurses, with support from a coordinator and supervisory personnel. (JB)

098   NR, NAP

Fraser, L. P. The reconstructed work week: One answer to the scheduling dilemma. In Warstler, M. E. (ed.) *Staffing: A Journal of Nursing Administration Reader.* Wakefield, Mass.: Contemporary Publishing, Inc., 1974. (See also #263)

Restructure of the work week by simultaneously altering the length of each shift and reducing the number of work days, combined with a simple two-week schedule cycle that alternates work periods of reasonable length (ten hours) with adequate rest periods, has proved successful. This rearrangement of the work week evenly distributes the staff over the seven days of a week and fulfills employee expectations without additional cost. The basic schedule was two weeks, MTFS of first week, SWTh of the second. Half the employees work the first shift, half the second shift. Under this work schedule, it is possible to assign a patient to one or the other of two complementary groups of employees rather than to a succession of constantly changing groups; this arrangement could facilitate continuity of care. (JB)

099   NR*

Frederickson, K. and Mayer, G. G. Problem solving skills: What effect does education have? *American Journal of Nursing.* July 1977, 77(7): 1167–1169.

Article based on an unpublished dissertation (D.Ed.) by the same authors, entitled "Problem-solving by nursing students: a twin study," Columbia University, Teachers College, New York City, 1974. An expanded framework on problem-solving was developed and became the basis for evaluating students. Students were shown a silent film which depicts five typical patient problems; three sequences were selected showing a woman about to have a radical mastectomy, a man experiencing an MI, and an elderly gentleman being admitted to the hospital. Responses of experts were categorized and became the basis for evaluating student responses. Fifty-five students in the last semester before graduation were tested, 28 from five BS programs and 27 from three AD programs. Each student was shown the films and her verbal responses recorded and later analyzed. Each student also completed a standardized test to assess general problem-solving (critical thinking) ability; the test was not specific to any field. Results: There was no significant difference in the process of problem-solving between the BS and AD students. The BS students did score significantly higher (p =.01) on the test of critical thinking. The authors note that the BS student did tend to score higher on the nursing problem series test. No evidence is presented regarding the validity or reliability of the film sequence as a measure of problem-solving. (JB)

100   NR*

Freund, L. E. *A model for measuring the difficulty of registered nurse-assignments.* (Doctoral dissertation, University of Michigan, 1969) Ann Arbor, Mich.: University Microfilms International, No. 69–18005.

The purpose of this research was to develop a model for measuring the difficulty of RN assignment. The model was validated by investigating the relationship between difficulty and performance in an experimental setting. The measures of performance were: the proportion of time spent by RNs in various kinds of activities and the proportion of a predefined set of activities which were successfully accomplished. The overall pattern of assignment was not considered in this study but is commented on in the literature review. During the estimation portion of the research, actual RN assignments were characterized according to the format required by the model. Using a scale of difficulty derived from a questionnaire administered to RNs, a difficulty value for each observed assignment

was obtained. Work sampling observations were grouped according to difficulty of assignment, while the average difficulty of assignments on a unit over a short period was associated with the proportion of activities from the completed checklist. Findings support the hypothesis that the computed measure of RN-assignment difficulty is significantly related to both the proportion of time spent in patient care activity and the proportion of nonpatient-oriented activities accomplished. There was significant indication that the average assignment difficulty reflects certain workload measures such as the number of RN hours per patient day and the number of RN hours per weighted patient day. There was also indication that the measure of assignment difficulty reflects the effects of using additional personnel on patient units with comparatively heavy workloads. These results imply the ability of the measure of assignment difficulty to be useful for characterizing the staff and workload situation on a patient unit in terms of a single variable, the average difficulty of RN assignments. (JC)

101   NAP, NR*

Freund, L. E. & Mauksch, I. G. *Optimal nursing assignments based on difficulty.* Final Project Report, USPHS, June 1975. Available from Medicus Affiliates, Inc., Evanston, Ill.

The approach taken in the difficulty methodology discussed in this paper is precisely the opposite to that of other staffing techniques. The assignments of personnel are structured first, based on required patient care activities, continuity constraints, and other factors until desirable assignments are reached. Staffing needs are then derived from examination of optimal solutions to the problem of structuring individual patient care assignments. The approach consists of building nursing assignments from a defined set of assignment elements which are viable in the model. Elements are defined for each nursing unit and reflect the way unit personnel structure and think about their assigments. A ratio scale reflecting the difficulty of each defined assignment element in relation to all other elements is obtained for each person or personnel type on the unit. This scale is only derived once for use in the assignment model and is updated thereafter only as technology, skills, or personnel change. The difficulty of any proposed assignment is computed by addition of the difficulties of the included assignment elements. Research results have documented the dependence of the time spent in patient care activities on the difficulty of RN, LPN, and technician assignments. Results also strongly support the relation of a process Quality Index to the average difficulty of personnel assignments; the relationship suggests optimum patient care quality is achieved at difficulty levels of 2.75 for RNs, 2.5 for LPNs, and 1.25 for aides. A computer model and supporting information system were developed for use with the system. The assignment heuristic achieves a very high degree of assignment balance between unit personnel. The solutions from the model differed significantly from head nurse and hospital staffing solutions. (Authors' abstract adapted)

102   NR

Friedman, P. & Schaur, I., et al. The IV laboratory nurse. *Hospitals.* September 16, 1972, 46(18): 102–107.

This article is a report on an innovation using nurses, instead of laboratory technicians, to perform venipunctures for the collection of laboratory specimens, as well as administration of intravenous fluids and blood transfusions. The team consisted of RNs and LPNs in a ratio of 4:1. (JC)

103   NR, NAP

Froebe, D. Scheduling: By team or individually. *Journal of Nursing Administration.* May-June 1974, 4(3):34–36.

Rotation of teams of airport control tower personnel are compared with the rotation of individuals within nursing services. The scheduling difference is cited as one reason for the small strides which have been achieved in applying small work group concepts into the delivery of nursing service at the unit level. The author notes some of the theoretical benefits of keeping a small work group's membership constant. (1) A correction mechanism within a team whose members are well-known to each other is an advantage in situations where the avoidance of errors is crucial. (2) Group cohesion results from consistent communication, which increases effectiveness. (3) Both competition and social support develop and foster creative prob-

lem solving by the group. (4) Decision making (about team members and schedules) may be placed close to its source of execution (the team unit). (JB)

104   NAP:TM, TPC

Gabbert, C. C. & Parkinson, J. Nursing utilization study, oncology station. In *The Patient Unit—Systems Approach.* Chicago, Ill.: Center for Hospital Management Engineering. American Hospital Associations, November 1974.

A nursing utilization study is rather disjointly described. The study's objectives were to determine nursing staffing requirements, including skill levels; provide data for scheduling which reflected patient care needs; evaluate operational aspects of the nursing station, including organization, procedures, layout, workload distribution, and personnel attitudes; document interdepartmental problems and aid in resolution; document, standardize, and distribute procedures; develop a management information system to monitor nurse utilization and aid planning of a float program; promote staff participation in management of the station. Partly describes change from team to TPC. (JB)

105   NR

Ganong, J. & Ganong, W. Are head nurses obsolete? *Journal of Nursing Administration.* September 1975, 5(7):16–18.

Discusses the role and functions of the head nurse. The authors conclude the role is essential; though the title may not be "head nurse," the role will necessarily be filled by persons with the same general responsibilities. They argue that there is no one best organization structure or role differentiation for every nursing department or organization. They encourage enrichment of the department of nursing service with a variety of roles as nursing meets its ever-increasing responsibilities and advise on expanded efforts to assist head nurses to become competent managers. (JB)

106   OS, NAP:TM

Garfield, S. R. An ideal nursing unit. *Hospitals.* June 16, 1971, 45(12):80–86.

The author writes about the "ideal nursing

unit" in terms of architectural design. Author cites studies that demonstrate that a linear work space form follows function, but not the organizational system of that function. The nature of "team nursing" is related to architectural structure. According to the author, the "team" consists of RNs, students, aides, orderlies, maids and clerks. It is obvious that the complete relationships involved in team nursing activities require a nearness to and visual awareness by team members of their leader and of each other. Linear designs hamper teamwork efficiency because form is not following function; it is fighting function. The basic form that facilitates team nursing is a visibly open circle. (JC)

107   PC, NR, NAP*:TM

George, F. L. & Kuehn, R. P. *Patterns of patient care*. New York: The Macmillan Company, 1955.

This volume reports a series of research studies designed to answer the following questions: (1) How much professional nursing service is required for medical-surgical patients in hospitals? (2) How much of what kind of nonprofessional nursing service is required? (3) How can the patients and nursing staff be organized into groups to provide the most effective care for each individual patient? (4) Can a staffing pattern be designed and demonstrated that will provide continuity of service for the patient and a balanced rotation of personnel from one tour of duty to another? Several chapters deal with the selection and training of clerks, aides, and LPNs. Factors to be considered in choosing an assignment pattern are discussed. In the chapter entitled "Designing the Group Pattern," the authors describe nine "patterns of nursing care" as well as comparisons of quality and satisfaction measures between these patterns as they were implemented. It appears that "team nursing" or "group nursing" is the NAP element in all patterns evaluated. The authors conclude that: (1) One professional nurse, one senior nurse aide and one junior nurse aide provided adequate nursing care for 12 to 16 patients on the day tour of duty. (2) One professional nurse and one junior nurse aide provided adequate service for 12 to 16 patients on the evening shift. (3) One professional nurse and one junior aide provided more service than could be utilized effectively on the night tour of duty for 24 to

32 patients. The remainder of the book addresses staffing methodologies. (JC)

108   PC, NR⁺, NAP:TM

Georgette, J. K. Staffing by patient classification. *Nursing Clinics of North America*. June 1970, 5(2):329–339.

Description of development and implementation of a patient classification system utilizing data from a Commission for Administrative Services in Hospitals (CASH) study to determine standard nursing hours required for certain tasks. There appears to be a "pool" from which nurses and assistants may be pulled to areas where they are needed, but description of this is vague. A "modified team nursing approach" was used with an LVN serving a functional role as "medication nurse." The author concludes that "staffing by patient classification is an assured and reliable method of providing adequate nursing care hours for a group of patients whose needs vary considerably. The system is flexible and allows for a large number of demanding patients or patients requiring minimal nursing care hours." (CAL)

109   NR*, OS*

Georgopoulos, B. S. *Hospital organization research: Review and source book*. Philadelphia: W. B. Saunders Co., 1974.

Review of empirical studies on hospital organization and intraorganizational relations in American hospitals by social-behavioral and administrative management investigators for the years 1960–1969. This is an excellent source book. (JB)

110   NR, OS, NAP:TM

Germaine, A. What makes team nursing tick. *Journal of Nursing Administration*. July-August 1971, 1(4):46–49.

Team nursing is defined as "a group of nurses working cooperatively toward a common goal, that of providing patient centered care . . . (This) differs from task-oriented care in that it focuses on the patient, not on the task." Reasons given for successful implementation include: (1) decentralized authority, (2) proper utilization of nurses, (3) environmental structure that keeps activity in the patients' rooms, (4) adequate services from hospital departments, and (5) support of medical staff and administration. (BK)

111   PC*

Gerson, L. W. Nursing care requirements—patient profiles of hospital care. *Canadian Hospitals.* September 1973, 50(9):49–53.

This paper reports the development of a technique of profiling the daily changes in the average amount of nursing care delivered to patients in various medical diagnostic categories. (JC)

112   NR*

Gorham, W. A. Staff nursing behaviors contributing to patient care and improvement. *Nursing Research.* Spring 1962, 11(2):68–79.

This research study concentrates on developing a comprehensive and systematic picture of the role of the general staff nurse. The critical incidence technique was used to collect data about the specific behaviors of general staff nurses which contribute to patient improvement. Questionnaires were given to staff nurses, supervisors and patients. A total of 2,065 incidences were classified into the following areas: I. Improving Patient's Adjustment to Hospitalization or Illness, II. Promoting Patient's Comfort and Hygiene, III. Contributing to Medical Treatment of Patient, IV. Arranging Management Details, and V. Personal Characteristics of the Nurse. In all 320 specific behaviors were listed under the categories. These lists of behaviors were given to 76 head nurses to determine the relative contributions of each of the categories of nursing behavior to the total job of patient care. The areas from the head nurse questionnaires are weighted in the following order of contribution (highest to lowest): contributing to medical treatment, arranging management details, improving patient's adjustment to hospitalization and treatment, promoting patient comfort and hygiene, personal characteristics. (JC)

113   OS*

Grady, R. An analysis of the effect that the unit manager has on the level of nursing activities at two major teaching university hospitals. (Un-

published master's thesis, The Ohio State University, 1974.) Available from University Microfilms International, Ann Arbor, Mich. *Abstracts of Hospital Management Studies,* No. 13766NU.

The purpose of this study was to determine if two alternate unit management systems produced any significant differences between the level of nursing activity on units at two large teaching hospitals. Unit #1 had a unit manager steadily present on the unit; Unit #2 had a unit manager available on an intermittent basis. The head nurse and staff RNs spent less time in administrative tasks on Unit #1 than on Unit #2. There were no significant differences in how LPNs spent their time on the units. It appeared from the results that the RNs spent the additional time in personal time, not in patient care time; the authors note the need to reorient the nurse to utilize the increased time available in patient care. (JC)

114   NAP⁺:TM

Grimm, C. Tradition yields to the nursing shortage. *Nursing Outlook.* August 1965, 13(8): 50–52.

Description of implementation of team nursing as a means to alleviate the problems of an almost insurmountable caseload, a continuing shortage of professional staff, and a high rate of turnover in the Bedford office of the VNA Brooklyn. (CAL)

115   NAP*, PC*

Gunter, L., Brantl, V., Esslinger, P. & Arndt, C. A study of three types of nursing assignments. *Nursing Research.* Winter 1964, 13(1):20–28.

This study was directed toward describing the nursing care activities of registered nurses in three types of assignments: special duty nursing, intensive care and staff nursing. Selected characteristics of patients grouped according to these assignments, and the nature of the nurse-client relationship was viewed by the nurse, with the purpose of identifying patterns of nursing care. It was concluded that fairly distinct patterns of care were associated with these three types of nursing assignments. The staff nursing assignment was characterized by emphasis on medications, treatments and procedures, and management activities for patients who were relatively physically independent and require a less active therapeutic regime. The special duty assignment was characterized by emphasis on individualized direct patient care for patients who require an active therapeutic regime and were physically dependent. The intensive care nursing assignment was characterized by emphasis on medications, treatments, and procedures and secondarily on direct patient care controlled by the nurse. (JC)

116   NAP*, NR, PC

Guthridge, F. E. An analysis of continuity of care as a function of the hospital system. (Unpublished masters thesis, University of Washington, School of Nursing, 1973.)

To achieve comprehensive health care the hospital system must facilitate the process of continuity of care. The structure and actions of the status-occupants within the system determine the outcome of the process of continuity of care. The purpose of the study was to identify and compare the actual observed structures and actions of the hospital system to those structures and actions anticipated, as described in the job specifications. Data were obtained by direct observation of the status-occupants on a medical unit over a 70-hour period of time. The observations were made in two-hour blocks of time, day and evening, from 7 A.M. until 9 P.M. Of 1,243 observations of the positions on the unit, only 67 behaviors could be related to fulfilling continuity of care needs of patients. Most of the continuity of care behaviors were done by the status-occupants in the Nurse Practitioner II position; most were done on the evening shift. The hospital system appeared dysfunctional to fulfilling the process of continuity of care because the position given the responsibility for initiating and completing referrals for continuing nursing care according to job specifications was not regularly assigned to the unit. (Abstracted in Western Interstate Commission for Higher Education in Nursing, *Newly Initiated and Completed Research,* Vol. 11, December 1975.)

117   NR, OS

Hagen, E. & Wolff, L. *Nursing leadership behavior in general hospitals.* New York: Institute of Research and Service in Nursing Education, Teachers College, Columbia University, 1961.

Descriptive study to determine the kinds of leadership behaviors displayed by head nurses, supervisors, and nursing service administrators in a general hospital setting, that are perceived by subordinates, peers, and superiors as facilitating or hindering the achievement of nursing service objectives in the hospital. Roles of various personnel, differences in hospitals, relationship of leadership to satisfaction and morale, and implications for basic and advanced educational and in-service programs as well as hospital organizational structure are discussed. (JB)

118   NR*

Hale, E. S. *Identification of the range of functions performed by graduates of associate degree nursing programs and graduates of baccalaureate degree nursing programs.* (Doctoral dissertation, University of Alabama, 1975) Ann Arbor, Mi.: University Microfilms International, No. 76–4816.

The purpose of this study was to identify the range of functions performed by graduates of associate degree nursing programs and graduates of baccalaureate degree programs. By examining nursing functions performed in planning nursing care for patients, it was anticipated that functions commonly performed by graduates of both types of nursing programs could be identified and differentiated. The three hypotheses tested in this study were: (1) There is no statistically significant difference between AD and BSN graduates in identifying nursing problems. (2) There is no statistically significant difference between AD and BSN graduates in stating care plan objectives. (3) There is no statistically significant difference between AD and BSN graduates in specifying nursing actions in the nursing care plan. Data were quantified in terms of number of correct responses to standardized patient descriptions and then analyzed via paired t-test or Chi-square. The effects of the employing hospitals on nursing care planning activities were not examined. Findings indicate the following: (1) The educational preparation of the two groups made no real difference in performance or identifying nursing problems. (2) Educational preparation of the two groups did associate with performance in stating objectives. Thirty percent of BSN graduates and 55 percent of AD graduates stated objectives unrelated to the nursing situation.

This difference was significant at the .05 level. (3) AD graduates stated more problems and more objectives which had no relationship to the nursing situation than BSN graduates. (4) BSN graduates more frequently than AD graduates reported daily or weekly preparation of written nursing care plans. (JC)

119   OS

Hanchett, E. *The problem oriented system: A literature review.* DHEW Pub. No. (HRA) 78-6, September 1977.

This bibliography was compiled as part of a study to design a method for determining the impact of the computerized problem-oriented record on the nursing components of patient care. The literature review is based on the system approach, which attempts to compare the nursing process approach and the problem-solving approach of the problem-oriented medical record system. The bibliography enhances the capability of determining the areas in which the problem-oriented record can assist, and the areas in which further development is required, in order to generate the information necessary for providing optimum care for the clients of nursing services. This is the third volume in the *Nurse Planning Information Series.* (From the Foreword by Jessie M. Scott.)

120   NR*, OS, NAP:CS, TM, FN

Harrington, H. A. & Theis, E. C. Institutional factors perceived by baccalaureate graduates as influencing their performance as staff nurses. *Nursing Research.* May-June 1968, 17(3):228–235.

The purpose of this study was to discover what are the perceptions of baccalaureate graduates in nursing who are employed at the Loeb Center as compared to those nurses employed in two typical hospitals. The questions the subjects were asked related to institutional conditions and requirements that help or hinder them in carrying out the functions of professional nursing. While nurses in typical (team/functional) settings identified factors in their work environment as deterrents, Loeb Center (case) nurses identified work factors as helpful in facilitating the carrying out of professional functions. Typical setting nurses noted that frequent change of assignment and multiple managerial and non-nursing tasks prevented continuity of patient care. Differences in attitudes of superiors and communication systems are also described. (JC)

121   OS⁺

Harris, C., Hawkins, W. F. & Markowich, M. M. Bigness doesn't have to mean poor communication. *Hospitals.* October 1, 1973, 47:56–62.

This article is a brief summary of a change project designed to improve communication between departments in a general hospital. In an effort to identify why the quality of care did not improve after increased expenditures, these authors uncovered the following: (1) The expansion of hospital facilities, patient volume and personnel led to greater reliance on written communication. (2) The functions of such new positions as nursing managers and team leaders were not adequately understood by all personnel. (3) The growth of specialization created impersonal professional relationships to the extent that many physicians did not know their patient's nurse. Described is an interdisciplinary committee which met weekly and recommended the following suggestions: (1) a more efficient system of assigning incoming patients to the appropriate rooms; (2) a regular time schedule for nurses to make rounds with physicians to assure face-to-face communication; (3) the practice of preadmission testing of all patients; (4) a program of group preoperative instruction; and (5) weekly teaching conferences for nursing staff taught by physicians. The conclusion was that this team approach improved patient care. No hard data was demonstrated. (JC)

122   PC

Hart, G. D. The I.V. nurse. *Hospital Administration in Canada.* October 1976, 18(10):62–64.

Advantages to patient care and the expanding role of the IV nurse are described. Benefits to particular patient groups are included. (JB)

123   PC*, NR*, OS*, NAP*:PN, TM, FN

Haussmann, R. K. D., Hegyvary, S. T. & Newman, J. F., Jr. *Monitoring quality of nursing care. Part II. Assessment and Study of Correlates.* DHEW Pub. No. (HRA) 76-7, July 1976. (See #139 for related monograph)

Report of the second phase of a contract let by DHEW's Division of Nursing to Rush-Presbyterian-St. Luke's Medical Center and Medicus Corporation. It describes a national trial of the quality-monitoring methodology, developed during the first phase of the contract, in 19 hospitals of differing size and characteristics. It reports relationships between the quality of the nursing process and a number of organizational and environmental factors, as well as exploration of the relationship between nursing process and patient outcome. Unit organizational structure was one of the variable sets significantly related to quality. Staff mix, size, coordination and care organization (NAP) had greater influence than staff attitudes and education. Leadership and staff satisfaction also contributed to quality. Excellent report. (JB)

124   OS⁺, NR

Hawkins, J. L. *The ward manager system: A case study of the organization of hospital nursing care.* (Doctoral dissertation, Purdue University, 1964) Ann Arbor, Mich.: University Microfilms International, No. 69–7410.

An intensive case study of a single ward was undertaken. It was studied before the ward manager was placed on the ward and then again three months later, after he had become established. A work sampling activities study and interaction study were performed before and after the change. A diary was kept by the ward manager. Casual and more structured observations were made. Questionnaire data were collected along with informal and semi-structured interviews. We found that a significant and substantial amount of the non-nursing administrative work formerly done by nurses was transferred to the ward manager with almost no resistance. However, there was no concomitant increase in the bedside care activities of the registered nurses despite the fact that they believed that they could have substantially increased their direct care time (and desired to do so). However, because of a very low ratio of registered nurses to other semi- and non-professional personnel, they felt constrained not to tie themselves down in patient care, but to remain free to manage and direct the bedside care given by others. In addition, the expectations of the remainder of role incumbents in the hospital social system remained unchanged and the nurses continued to receive most of the

requests and demands for coordinative-administrative activity, although they turned most of the actual work over to the ward manager. Responding to these expectations caused the nurse to spend much time simply being "accessible" near the nurses' station. Finally, the reward structure of the hospital worked in such a way as to promote the nurses' activity in administrative affairs at the expense of nursing care. (Author's abstract)

125   NAP

Hegyvary, S. T. Foundations of primary nursing. *Nursing Clinics of North America.* June 1977, 12(2):187–196.

This paper explores first the organization of nursing care in the past (functional, team) and some of the factors that have influenced changes in directions. Then the concept of primary nursing is discussed, including findings from studies of primary nursing (satisfaction, quality, cost). (CAL)

126   OS*

Hegyvary, S. T. & Chanings, P. A. The hospital setting and patient care outcomes. *Journal of Nursing Administration.* Part I: March-April 1975, 5(3):29–32. Part II: May 1975, 5(4):36–42.

A study of the effects of preoperative stress, provision of preoperative instructions, and hospital setting on postoperative outcomes is described. In Part II, the findings are presented; they indicate that hospital setting was the only consistently significant variable. The authors consider the possibility that a patient-centered philosophy, open leadership style, and effective coordination among departments allowed the beneficial effects of preoperative instruction and resulting patient understanding to appear by facilitating postoperative behaviors that would prevent complications. (JB)

127   NR

Hellman, C. The making of a clinical specialist. *Nursing Outlook.* March 1974, 22(3):165–167.

This article describes the issues in establishing the role of a clinical nursing specialist of a single person in a large university medical center. Problems identified were: (1) lack of a role model, (2) setting priorities and limitations, (3) lack of structure for the role within the organization, (4) performance evaluation, and (5) producing effective change. (JC)

128   PC, NAP⁺:CS

Henderson, C. Can nursing care hasten recovery? *American Journal of Nursing.* 1964, 64:80–83.

Nursing care is the treatment at Loeb Center—a unique facility where professional nurses are "back at the bedside" helping patients by means of a new approach. They are testing the theory that patients beyond the crisis-therapy state will go home sooner when they are cared for wholly by professional nurses. A report of Loeb Center's first 14 months of operation. (CAL)

129

Horn, B. J. Personal communication. 1977.

Information collected from interviews of hospital personnel during previous studies by the author. (JB)

130   OS, NR, NAP

Horn, B. J. & Parker, J. C. Reorganization of nursing resources in hospitals. Unpublished manuscript, 1975.

Description of the changes in nursing roles in 19 nursing service departments, including the preconditions and design principles required for successful change. Changes are described within the context of four basic components of nursing care: comprehensiveness, continuity, accountability, and coordination. Assignment patterns are described. (JC)

131   OS⁺

Howe, G. E. Decentralization aids coordination of patient care services. *Hospitals.* March 1, 1969, 43(5):53–56.

This author reports that decentralized patient care administration allows departmental directors to fulfill their responsibilities for education, research, and policy development, rather than being tied down to numerous operating prob-

lems. In order to alleviate the problems created by the vertical growth of departments in a large and expanding hospital, the hospital was divided into component parts. Eight distinct patient areas were determined: medical care, surgical care, operating room care, OB care, pulmonary disease care, psychiatric care, physical medicine and rehabilitation care, and ambulatory care. Each of these areas was then organized along the lines of a separate hospital with its own administrator. The effects of the decentralized reorganization on nursing personnel were: (1) Lines of communication were exceedingly short. (2) The director of nursing gained the most because it provided her the chance to grow and gain in importance to the hospital and the nursing profession. NAP used at this agency was "team" nursing prior to and following implementation of decentralized administration of services. (JC)

132   NR*

Hurka, S. J. Organizational environment and work satisfaction. *Dimensions in Health Service.* January 1974, 51(1):41–43.

Study dealing with job satisfaction among registered nurses in hospitals, public health agencies, and educational institutions. A questionnaire was used to gather data, and results were calculated by simple correlations. The findings were: (1) Nurses with higher educational qualifications (baccalaureate degree) and more lengthy preparation prefer to work in a nonhospital setting. A large proportion of nurses working in hospitals possessed a diploma degree in nursing. (2) Nursing education and public health agencies tend to attract older nursing personnel. Requirements for higher educational qualifications, longer work experience, maturity, preference for day work, and absence of organizational factors (rules, regulations and limits of authority) help to explain the tendency for older nurses to enter these two types of organizations. (3) Organizational environment is related to job satisfaction of nurses. The findings in this study indicate a higher degree of job satisfaction for nurses working in nursing education and public health compared to nurses working in hospitals. (4) The response to the questions dealing with career orientation indicates there is no relationship between organizational environment and perceived satisfaction with nursing as a career. (JPK)

134   NAP⁺:PN

Isler, C. Rx for a sick hospital: Primary nursing care. *RN*. February 1976, 39(2):60–65.

Description of implementation of primary nursing assignment pattern, reported one year after primary nursing was put in operation. The benefits of this NAP ("an unqualified success") include increased bed occupancy, markedly diminished nurse turnover rate, high staff morale, virtually no absenteeism, cost effectiveness, and increased patient satisfaction. The nursing staff held a two-day conference reporting on the success of their project and planned to participate in two national conferences on primary nursing care in April and May 1976. (CAL)

135   PC, NR, OS*

Jaco, E. G. Evaluation of nursing and patient care in a circular and rectangular hospital unit—final report. A report to Hill Family Foundation, 1967. Available from E. Gartley Jaco, Ph.D., Department of Sociology, University of California, Riverside, California 92502.

Final report on a study which quantitatively evaluated the effects of physical design on patient care and efficiency in the use of nursing personnel in a general hospital. Phase I compared patients needing intermediate care, Phase II patients requiring intensive care and Phase III self-care patients. Ten dependent variables were investigated: type, amount and level of nursing care; nurses' utilization of unit; patient welfare; patient satisfaction; nursing staff satisfaction; physician satisfaction; length of stay; and costs of patient care. Twelve study situations were set up for each level of care in which occupancy and nursing staff levels were varied. The report gives results when all study situations are pooled as well as individual findings for each study situation. Some of the major findings are: (1) In situations where there is a high demand for patient care and a limited nursing staff, the circular unit has more advantages in providing total patient care than the angular unit. (2) Some types of patients are not suitable for a circular unit. (3) The circular unit is designed more for staff convenience than patient convenience. (4) Reducing demands for patient care is more detrimental to the morale of nursing staff on a circular unit than an angular

unit. (5) Operational costs are less for circular unit in size studies (22 beds) with equal or better quality patient care than angular unit. It is concluded that physical design can lower costs without impairing quality of care depending on psychological, administrative, medical, and social utilization of the unit. (D.F.B.) (From *Abstracts in Hospital Management Studies*, June 1968, 4:161.)

136   PC, NR*, OS

Jagla, B. A. Stress factors identified by nurses in the intensive care unit. (Unpublished master's thesis, University of California, Los Angeles, 1975.)

The purpose of this study was to identify those factors in the Intensive Care Unit (ICU) that nurses reported as stressful. Though the stressful factors in the ICU and related effects on the ICU nurse had been mentioned in articles, there was no documented research. A methodological and descriptive evaluative survey was done. Data were obtained through a written questionnaire. Forty-six female registered nurses who had worked longer than six months in the ICU participated in the study. These nurses functioned as full-time staff members in the ICU and had no administrative duties. Six hospitals in the greater Los Angeles and Orange County areas were used for data collection. ICU nurses identified specific factors occurring in the ICU as stressful. The factors were derived from the four categories of stressful factors and their sixteen components. The categories and their components are as follows: (1) Interpersonal—(a) communication problems between staff and physicians, (b) communication problems between staff and nursing office, (c) communication problems between staff members, (d) communication problems between staff and other departments in the hospital; (2) Environmental—(a) numerous equipment and its failure, (b) physical injury to the nurse, (c) physical setup of the ICU, (d) noise level in the ICU; (3) Patient Care—(a) work load and amount of physical work required, (b) meeting the psychological needs of the patient, (c) meeting the needs of the family, (d) death of the patient; (4) Knowledge Base—(a) patient teaching, (b) cardiac arrest, (c) amount of rapid decisions that must be made in the ICU, (d) amount of knowledge needed to work in the ICU. In regard to main categories of stress factors, Patient Care was viewed as the highest stress factor while Knowledge Base was shown to be the lowest. Analysis of components indicated work load and amount of physical work required as the highest stress factor, death of the patient second, communication problems between the staff and the nursing office third, and communication problems between staff and physicians as fourth in degree of perceived stress factors. In the reverse order, patient teaching was scored as the least stressful component, cardiac arrest next, communication problems between staff and other departments in the hospital third, and meeting the psychological needs of the patient as fourth. Age, level of nursing education, years of general nursing experience and years of experience in the ICU were found not to be significantly correlated with the stress factor scores of the subjects. Additionally, a significant correlation was not obtained between nurses who had worked less than six months in the ICU. The findings of this study indicated specific factors in the ICU that were stressful to the nurse. Recommendations for nursing administration, hospital in-service education, schools of nursing, and future nursing research were cited. (Abstract from Western Interstate Commission on Higher Education in Nursing, *Newly Initiated and Completed Research,* Vol. 11, December 1975)

137   NR*, OS*

Jarratt, V. R. *A study of conceptions of autonomous nursing actions appropriate for the staff nurse role.* (Unpublished doctoral dissertation, University of Texas, Austin, June 1967.)

This well-done descriptive survey resulted in the following conclusions: (1) Conflicts in expectations for autonomous action in the staff nurse role were found to exist among the significant groups who influence the role—senior nursing students, instructors, head nurses and supervisors, staff nurses, and physicians. (2) Consensus among groups, on the whole, exists for actions that can be regulated, or are apt to be regulated, by procedures and policies. On the other hand, differences tend to increase within and among groups in expectations for actions requiring individualized nursing judgement and evaluation of needs. (3) Considerable role confusion and ambiguity about the autonomous areas of nursing seem to exist among these groups. (4) Nursing service personnel tend to

expect a more traditionally dependent role for the nurse than instructors and students do. (5) The scope and nature of autonomy perceived as appropriate for the staff nurse increases in relation to the educational level attained. Other relationships among the groups and implications for education and administration are described. (JB)

138   PC, NR

Jelinek, R. C. *Nurse scheduling control system.* Available from University Microfilms International, Ann Arbor, Mich. *Abstracts of Hospital Management Studies,* No. NU1199.

Detailed description of a generalized procedure for decision making in the allocation of available personnel to individual patient units. The program gives consideration to two criteria in achieving an optimum utilization of available personnel: to allocate personnel according to workload and to minimize changes in personnel assignments. It also gives consideration to substitutability of one personnel category for another, preference of personnel regarding floating, and administration's desires to restrict assignments of individual personnel. (JB)

139   PC

Jelinek, R. C., Haussmann, R. K. D., Hegyvary, S. T. & Newman, J. F. *A methodology for monitoring quality of nursing care.* Bureau of Health Manpower, Division of Nursing, DHEW Pub. No. (HRA) 76-25, July 1975. (see #123 also)

Report of the activities and results of the first twelve months of a project to develop a methodology for monitoring quality of nursing care. The methodology which was developed is based on a master criteria list of 239 criteria grouped under 28 subobjectives within 6 objectives for the process of nursing care, available for use on medical, surgical, pediatric and related intensive care units. It incorporates all useful criteria in existing methodologies, is internally statistically consistent and reliable, economically feasible, and permits ready inclusion of future research results. A unified conceptual framework of the nursing process and model of the patient care system are described in the section (III) on methodology development. Patient classification is also discussed, in Appendix A. (JB)

140   OS

Jelinek, R. C., Munson, F. & Smith, R. L. *SUM: An organizational approach to improved patient care.* Battle Creek, Mi.: W. K. Kellogg Foundation, February 1971.

This study was done to evaluate whether Service Unit Management reduced costs, improved quality of care, saved professional nursing time, increased personnel satisfaction, and set a stage for further improvements, as claimed. Findings concluded that SUM neither reduced nor significantly increased personnel costs, was effective in relieving nursing of responsibility for many nonnursing activities, allowed higher quality of patient care and more efficient functioning on units, resulted in higher job satisfaction of nurses, and provided opportunities for additional important changes. Characteristics of unit management programs, including tasks and responsibilities assigned to SUM, its focus, organizational structure, qualifications of personnel, and the change process in implementation are described. The report is based on a two and one-half year study in eight hospitals (total of 55 patient units) combined with a national questionnaire survey. An annotated bibliography is included. (JB)

141   PC*

Johnson, J. E., Rice, V. H., Fuller, S. S. & Endress, P. M. Sensory information, instruction in a coping strategy, and recovery from surgery. *Research in Nursing and Health.* 1978, 1(1):4-17.

Instruction in a specific coping strategy and information about events and sensations had beneficial effects for cholecystectomy patients but had only minor effects for herniorrhaphy patients. (JB)

142   PC, NR

Johnson, M. M. & Martin, H. W. A sociological analysis of the nurse role. In Skipper, J. K. & Leonard, R. C. *Social Interaction and Patient Care.* Philadelphia: J. B. Lippincott Company, 1965.

From a sociological viewpoint, the authors describe the expressive function as the nurse's

specialized function as a professional person, equally important to the social system as the instrumental and technical functions of the physician. The activities of the nurse in caring are seen as providing for tension release for patients in the stressful situation of being ill and hospitalized, and also in providing a harmonious, integrated relationship between the physician, nurse, and patient. (JB)

143   NR*, OS*

Johnston, R. Nurses and job satisfaction. A review of some research findings. *Australian Nurses' Journal.* May 1976, 5(11):23-27.

In a review of some research findings relative to the growing concern over the number of nurses leaving the profession, pertinent findings of five studies were presented concerning job dissatisfaction of nurses in Great Britain, the United States, Canada, and Australia. The need for better economic and working conditions was well documented, yet claims for higher salaries were seen by some researchers as an expression of frustrations in many other aspects of the work situation. The expected dedication and selfless service of nurses appeared marred by community exploitation of this involvement along with discriminatory and unsatisfactory relationships with supervisors, medical staff (status of nurses), and other hospital personnel. In delineating job disadvantages and other related factors, the competence and quality of supervision, understood in its widest sense, was found to be paramount for job satisfaction. Each researcher included recommendations and suggestions for improvement in the working conditions of nurses, yet warned against simplified explanations for nurses' dissatisfactions with their jobs. (Abstract from *Nursing Research,* Jan.-Feb. 1977, 26(1):73.)

144   PC

Jones, E. W. *Patient classification for long-term care: User's manual.* DHEW Pub. No. (HRA) 75-3107, November 1974.

Tool developed, on the basis of four research projects on long-term care, and field-tested. Usable for multiple purposes, including planning staffing allocation. (JB)

145   PC, NAP*:PN

Jones, K. Study documents effect of primary nursing on renal transplant patients. *Hospitals.* December 16, 1975, 49(24):85–89.

A study was conducted by the author at University Medical Center, Ann Arbor, to evaluate the effect of primary nursing on the postoperative adaptation of renal transplant patients. The nursing staffs of two hospital units involved in the care of kidney transplant patients participated in this study, with several regular staff members volunteering to function as primary nurses. From her results, the author arrived at the following conclusions: patients respond to major surgical intervention more quickly and with fewer problems if one nurse is responsible for planning and managing their care throughout their hositalization; nurses can be instrumental in reducing the cost of hospitalization by facilitating early recovery after surgery and earlier discharge from hospital confinement; patients respond well to personalized care and to having a familiar nurse caring for them rather than different nurses every few days or, in some cases, every day. (CAL)

146   NAP⁺:TM

Joy, Patricia M. Maintaining continuity of care during shift change. *Journal of Nursing Administration.* November-December 1975, 5(9):28–29.

Centering the change of shift activity about "patient rounds" provided the opportunity to assess and evaluate patient care, improved communication between nursing shifts and between nurses and patients. Continuity of care was enhanced. (JB)

147

Kaluzny, A. D. Innovation in health services: Theoretical framework and review of research. *Health Services Research.* Summer 1974, 9(2): 101–120.

The arrangements comprising the health care delivery system are analyzed in terms of social organization, and selected characteristics of the system are discussed that are pertinent to the study of diffusion and adoption of various types of innovations. Research currently under way or completed is then reviewed in terms of its contribution to overall understanding of the phenomenon of innovation on both the individual practitioner and the organizational levels. The analysis is then used to delineate problem areas needing further study. The article provides a useful context in which to consider substantive findings of future empirical research. (Author's abstract)

148   OS⁺

Kauffman, S. H. Unit management: A twelve year appraisal. *Hospitals.* August 1, 1975, 49(15): 67–71.

This somewhat informal article presents problems encountered by a hospital in implementing unit management. (JC)

149   NAP*⁺:TM

Kelly, P. A. & Lambert, K. L. The effect of a modified team approach on nurse-patient interaction and job satisfaction. *Journal of Nursing Administration.* April 1978, 8(4):3–9.

In a year-long experiment on one hospital unit, the team nursing approach was refined: permanent team leaders were named, and members were assigned to each team on a permanent basis. At various intervals throughout the project, team personnel were questioned regarding job satisfaction, and patients were questioned regarding their perception of the nursing care they received. The results were not conclusive, due in part to difficulties encountered in implementing the assignment pattern. A major difficulty was lack of real understanding of the objectives by the participants and alterations in the study design. Results were: (1) failure to demonstrate the team leader position as a clinical leadership position; (2) inability to document the effect on implementation of the plan of care, although planning for patient care improved; (3) communication among team members did not improve, but communication with patients and families was substantially enhanced; (4) stability of nurse-patient interaction did not occur, and job satisfaction of staff did not increase; (5) patients' knowledge of their illness and discharge planning increased; their ability to identify staff caring for them increased. The validity (as an administrative system) of the staffing pattern was not demonstrated, due in part to change in staffing procedures midway through the project. The authors recommend attention to change process and validation of participants' understanding in future projects of this nature. (JB)

150   PC

Key, G. A. Categorization of patients according to their needs for nursing care. (Unpublished master's thesis, University of Toronto, School of Hygiene, 1971.) Available from University Microfilms International, Ann Arbor, Mich. *Abstracts of Hospital Management Studies,* No. NUO-8381.

A matrix was developed of "every conceivable (including psychosocial and teaching) patient need" for a point system of classification. The matrix was too cumbersome for actual implementation but was used as basis for further development by a local hospital. (JB)

151   NR, NAP:TM, PN[+]

Kilpack, V. The head nurse creates a new order for clinical learning. *Journal of Nursing Administration.* October 1976, 6(8):41–46.

A young head nurse capable of making ideas turn to action, engaged her staff and baccalaureate students in structuring a climate for care that harmonized with the most current directives for nursing practice. Her leadership improved the effectiveness of team nursing and eventually resulted in a change over to primary nursing. (JB)

152   OS, NR, NAP*[+]:PN

Knecht, A. A., Marram, G. & Schlegel, M. Innovation on four tower west. *American Journal of Nursing.* May 1973, 73(5):808–816.

Three articles on an experiment in innovative nursing on a unit staffed by new graduates. The nurses selected primary nursing as the assignment pattern for the unit. The articles describe why and how the experiment was initiated, and what happened. Graduates on the experimental unit maintained high professional ideals and demonstrated high job satisfaction compared with new graduates on other units. Cost and patient satisfaction were equivalent to the control units. (JB)

153

Kovner, A. R. *The nursing unit: A technological perspective.* (Doctoral dissertation, University of Pittsburgh, School of Public and International Affairs, 1966.) Available from University Microfilms International, Ann Arbor, Mich. *Abstracts of Hospital Management Studies,* No. NU1018.

This study examines unit organization from the perspective of organizational theory and is primarily useful in its theoretical framework and hypotheses. The author proposes that the technology of nursing units varies according to the variability of patients and the predictability of techniques. He suggests that patients be assigned to units according to the nursing technology predicted for their care, that nurses be allocated by grade to the new units, and that differences in structure (e.g. supervision) should parallel the differences in the unit technology and personnel. He outlines hospital opposition and physical layout constraints. The author does a descriptive study of the technology and variability/predictability variables in six hospitals and the analysis of the results appears to support his hypotheses. Unfortunately, however, the measures of technology are primarily task-oriented and exhibit a medical model orientation that casts some doubt on their accuracy and validity for nursing. Similar problems and questionable assumptions also cast doubt on the measures of variability and predictability. The study has promising theoretical propositions, but they need to be retested in the light of clearer presentations of nursing practice theory and patient variables. (JB)

154   NAP[+]:CS

Kowalski, K. E. On call staffing. *American Journal of Nursing.* October 1973, 73(10):1725–1727. (See also #219)

This article describes a staffing pattern incorporating "teams of nurses"—two nurses in each. Throughout a patient's pregnancy, she sees both team nurses in the prenatal clinic and one or both nurses in the labor and delivery suite, the postpartum unit, and the nursery. The author contends that this system alleviates fragmentation of care. The over-all staffing pattern consists of four teams of two nurses who care for clinic patients and eight nurses who are scheduled on a traditional staffing pattern. Each two-nurse team carries a case load of clinic patients representing about 25–30 deliveries per month. (JC)

155   PC, NR, NAP*⁺:TM

Kraegel, J. M. *An integrated systems approach to meeting patient needs.* Available from Center for Hospital Management Engineering, American Hospital Association, Chicago, December 1973.

Description of restructuring of patient care system and demonstration experiment; the patient care system was based on patient needs, and all designs were related to making the care system effective, with efficiency a secondary consideration. A 39-bed medical-surgical unit was the demonstration unit. The nursing assignment pattern involved work groups, called "flights," which were assigned to small groups of patients. The personnel were assigned according to skill level required to perform tasks required by patients. Continuity of personnel in the work group was maintained as much as possible, especially the leader. RNs were assigned as leaders and had responsibility for care, but they actively involved flight members in planning. Care plans were highly visible. Most of the RNs were diploma graduates. The independent variable, patient care system design, included four subsystems in the demonstration unit test: medications, materials supply, communication, and plan of care. (Other subsystems were elements of the design but were not tested.) The dependent variables were: cost, number of personnel needed, workload, patient care quality. Quality measures included patient care planning, time spent with patients, and patient satisfaction. Cost measures included absenteeism. Job satisfaction of nurses was also measured. Instruments included personnel questionnaires, C.A.S.H. Quality Control Index, patient classification and activity study, and patient satisfaction indexes. Information about methodology and tools is not given except that it was an evaluation of the demonstration unit by Medicus Corporation. Results indicated no increase in costs or personnel were necessary. The demonstration unit carried one and one-half times the workload of the control unit. Better patient care planning and higher patient satisfaction were also demonstrated; all levels of nursing personnel on the demonstration unit spent twice as much time with patients as nursing personnel on the control unit. Nurse job satisfaction was higher on the demonstration unit and absenteeism was reduced. (JB)

156   NAP:TM

Kramer, M. Team nursing—a means or an end? *Nursing Outlook.* 1971, 19(10):648–652.

The author interviewed directors of nursing service in 37 medical center hospitals in the United States as part of an ongoing research program; questions were asked regarding team spirit, methods of assignment, and team conferences. This article compares the means-end focus of team nursing from its early conception to its present operation and also assesses the current state of team nursing practice, on the basis of observations and interviews with nursing service directors, inservice educators, and nurse practitioners (i.e., staff nurses). (CAL)

157   NAP⁺:TM

Kron, T. *Nursing team leadership.* 2nd edition. Philadelphia: W. B. Saunders, 1966.

The objectives of this second edition are to bring information up to date and to include more information about activities important in the effective practice of team leadership. Definitions and discussions of nursing care, team nursing, and leadership are included. How to organize work, supervise the team, conduct conferences, use nursing care plans, and relate to others in the hospital are also discussed. The book is directed toward helping the professional nursing student prepare for her role as team leader. (JC)

158   NAP:TM

Kron, T. Team nursing—how viable is it today? *Journal of Nursing Administration.* Nov.-Dec. 1971, 1(6):19–22.

Author states that team nursing, to be viable, must place emphasis on (1) the importance of leadership by the registered nurse in planning and giving nursing care and (2) adequate communication to insure continuity of planned individualized patient care. (BK)

159 PC

Laberge-Nadeau, C. & M. F. A simulation study of nursing staff utilization. *Canadian Hospital.* May 1972, 49(5):54–57.

A study was undertaken at this childrens' hospital to: (1) classify patients according to their needs and attempt to determine the amount of care required, and (2) study the tasks of types of nursing personnel in order to reorganize and reassign them to maximize the efficiency of each group. The discussion of methodology and results is done in a rather confusing fashion. Requirements for care are viewed as either direct care of patients or nondirect care. The authors conclude that nondirect care is independent of the number and class of patients under normal conditions. Response to direct care needs may entail a better distribution of tasks between personnel categories and/or the addition of staff. Apparently, some form of team nursing was being used. Patients were categorized into four classes of care requirements (I. Minimum, II. Moderate, III. Acute, IV. Intensive) on the basis of their needs for independence, physical and psychological support, ambulation, observation and surveillance, and other specific nursing needs or treatment. (JB)

160 NR, NAP⁺:TM

Lambertson, E. *Nursing team organization and functioning.* New York: Teachers College, Columbia University, 1953.

Written as a guide to team organization and functioning, based on the first studies of team organization and the experience of the author, this report describes in detail the structure and roles of the nursing team, its relationship to other health personnel, the education and preparation of leaders and team members, and implementation of the system in hospitals. (JB)

161 PC, OS⁺

LaMontagne, M. E. & McKeehan, K. M. Profile of a continuing care program emphasizing discharge planning. *Journal of Nursing Administration.* October 1975, 5(8):22–33.

This article describes the approach of one hospital in developing a systematic approach to coordinating patient needs with available resources in the community. Evaluation showed impressive increases in the hospital's referrals to community agencies, positive responses from hospital staff and agencies involved. The guidelines for implementation are listed and the implementation of each is discussed. The program is hospital-based and uses a multidisciplinary team approach. (JB)

162 NAP:PN

Leonard, M. Health issues and primary nursing in nephrology care. *Nursing Clinics of North America.* September 1975, 10(3):413–420.

A "think piece" describing why primary nursing is the ideal model for delivery of patient care in nephrologic settings. Some of the reasons cited are cost effectiveness, increased responsibility and professional accountability, improved quality of patient care, and increased nurse and patient satisfaction. Many observations are presented, e.g., "special orientation programs and serious leadership support are necessary," but no concrete examples from experience are given. (CAL)

163 NR, OS

Levine, E., ed. *Research in nurse staffing in hospitals.* DHEW Pub. No. (NIH) 73–434, 1973. (See also a companion volume, by M. Aydelotte, #014.)

Report of the Conference on Research on Nurse Staffing in Hospitals, sponsored by the Division of Nursing in Fredericksburg, Va., May 23–25, 1972. An overview of nurse staffing research. Papers presented on variables considered to be significant in influencing the quantitative and qualitative demand for nurse staffing are included. Variables addressed include patients' requirements for nursing services, architectural design of the hospital, administrative and cost factors, and social psychological factors. Papers were also presented on the evaluation of quality of nursing care and the impact of computerized information systems on staffing. Presentations for discussion and task force reports are included. The report contains findings on important areas of research into nurse staffing, identifies gaps in the existing knowledge, and suggests future directions. (Adapted from the Introduction)

164   PC, NR*, OS

Levine, H. D. & Phillip, P. J. *Factors affecting staffing levels and patterns of nursing personnel.* DHEW Pub. No. (HRA) 75–6, February 1975.

Data from four sources were used to analyze the employment of nursing personnel in community hospitals from the perspectives of demand, need, and potential of hospital care for the community. Regression models were developed for each of six personnel categories based on the consideration of 21 independent variables, including variables describing the facilities and services of the hospital, other organizational and product characteristics, socioeconomic characteristics of the area, demographic characteristics of the population, and personnel supply characteristics. The hospital models were stratified as nonprofit/nonteaching, nonprofit/teaching, and profit types; 3,800 hospitals provide the data base. The analyses provide new perspectives for looking at the distribution of nursing personnel. (JB)

165   NAP:TM

Lio, A. M. Leadership and responsibility in team nursing. *Nursing Clinics of North America.* June 1973, 8(2):267–281.

This article attempts to tell how one hospital restructured the organization of nursing service to facilitate the preparation of nurses for leadership roles as "team" leaders. Problems in clinical competence, delegation of authority, and limitations within a hierarchical organization are mentioned but not explored in any depth. Issues in nursing education are highlighted in terms of preparing practitioners not ready for the realities of nursing practice. The head nurse is defined as the coordinator of patient care. Suggestions are directed to nurse educators. The article does not present any empirical basis for conclusions. (JC)

166

Lippitt, G. L. Hospital organization in the post-industrial society. *Hospital Progress.* June 1973, 54:55–64.

Hospital organizational structures and processes which conform to those of the industrial era will be neither effective nor acceptable in the changing environment of the post-industrial era. Nine characteristics of the hospital organization in the future and their implications for hospital administrators are discussed in this article, as are the social, philosophical, and psychological forces which will influence change. Key characteristics of the future organization: (1) Hospitals will require new structures to cope with needed flexibility in health care needs. (2) Development of human resources will become a key responsibility of future organizations. (3) Mutual confidence, rather than obedience to authority, will provide the basis of work accomplishment. (4) Freedom of access to information and two-way communication will characterize the system. (5) Increased interface between state, local, and federal government with private and public institutions will create opportunities and problems. (6) There will be both increased centralization and decentralization of decision-making areas throughout the organization. (7) Conflict, confrontation, and stress will continue as a norm of organizational life. (8) Effective face-to-face groups will be the key unit of organizational accomplishment. (9) General system concepts will be utilized and applied in organizations. (JB)

167   NR*

Longest, B. B. Jr. Job satisfaction for registered nurses in the hospital setting. *Journal of Nursing Administration.* May-June 1974, 4(3):46–52.

A comparison is made between responses from 195 RNs from ten Atlanta hospitals to questions about job satisfaction and the classic study by Frederick Herzberg on job satisfaction. Nursing educators in the State of Georgia were also queried, and their responses were compared to those of practicing RNs. The conclusions may benefit nursing administrators who must deal with problems of turnover, absenteeism, and productivity among RNs. The article provides a potentially helpful, though brief, literature review on studies of job satisfaction and describes an easily administered questionnaire. (JB)

168   PC, NAP⁺

Lunt, J. Bridging the gap in continuity of care. *Nursing Times.* March 19, 1970, 66:372.

Improved continuity of care and service to patients has resulted since a district nursing liaison arrangement was established between a hospital and three local authorities. The arrangement enables the nursing liaison officer to: (1) Make hospital ward rounds each morning with the medical and nursing staff of the hospital, thus improving the understanding between them. (2) Visit the patient while still in the hospital. This has lessened the patient's anxiety about aftercare, and it gives the nurse the opportunity to assess the patient's requirements for home care. (3) Visit the home on the day of operation—to reassure relatives and tell them about postoperative care. Since the establishment of this two-way service, the staff public health nurse feels more comfortable about calling the hospital and obtaining certain services or changes in services for her patients as the need arises, e.g., rescheduling outpatient appointments, delaying hospital discharges, or obtaining hospital readmission. (JB)

169   PC, NAP+:FN

Lyons, J. P. & Young, J. P. A staff allocation model for mental health facilities. *Health Services Research.* Spring 1976, 11(1):53–68.

This article describes a model for allocating staff within a large psychiatric hospital. It provides an objective framework within which one can test alternating staff operating policies before making critical decisions concerning the employment of one category of personnel as opposed to another. It is based on objective data describing patient needs and staff functioning patterns. Besides being useful for short-term deployment of staff and budgetary resources, it can also be used as a long-range planning tool for testing modifications in policy decisions and budget proposals. The algorithm employed, mixed-integer linear programming, is readily available; computer costs and running time are relatively minimal. The basis of the model concerns the appropriate assignment of personnel to therapeutic activities; assumptions are stated explicitly. (JB)

170   NR*, OS*

Lyons, T. F. Nursing attitudes and turnover: The relation of social-psychological variables to turnover, propensity to leave, and absenteeism among hospital staff nurses. Available from University Microfilms International, Ann

Arbor, Mich. *Abstracts of Hospital Management Studies,* No. NU1150.

A study of certain organizational and individual factors for nurses' turnover and absenteeism. The study was limited to community general hospitals (300–499 beds) at two levels of analysis: individual and organization. Two samples were used: the national sample—for purposes of study other than turnover, and an intensive sample—for data from nurses within one hospital. The conditions affecting withdrawal positively or negatively were job satisfaction, tensions, role clarity and communication. Data in the national sample were collected from questionnaires administered to 149 registered nurses in ten hospitals. Data in the intensive sample were collected from questionnaires completed by 217 staff nurses of one hospital who were employed during 1965, including those who left during 1965, and including those who left during the period. "Affective variables, cognitions, and perceptions of organizational functioning were found to be related to voluntary nursing withdrawal, and were also found to be interrelated." "Immediate supervision was not found to be a factor consistently related to withdrawal." (L.E.W.) (From *Abstracts of Hospital Management Studies,* June 1969, V:142.)

171   PC, NAP+:CS

Mass, M. L. Nurse autonomy and accountability in organized nursing services. *Nursing Forum.* 1973, 12(3):237–259. (See #172 also)

The purpose of this article was to theoretically analyze nurse autonomy and accountability as necessary means for improved patient care. A program to improve patient welfare at a long-term care facility in Iowa was used to illustrate how professional nurse autonomy and accountability can evolve and be used to improve care of patients within a bureaucratic institution. (CAL)

172   PC, NAP+:CS

Mass, M., Specht, J. & Jacox, A. Nurse autonomy: Reality, not rhetoric. *American Journal of Nursing.* December 1975, 75(12):2201–2208. (See #171 also)

A group of nurses at the Iowa Veteran's Home developed a professional model of practice within a bueaucratic organization. A number of factors contributed to their decision to begin this process: the setting, the philosophy and leadership of the nursing director, and the opportunity to grow together as they participated in decisions regarding nursing practice. This article describes the evolution of the philosophy behind their nursing practice, the conceptualization of their professional model, and the development of collective authority and accountability in an effort to improve patient welfare. (CAL)

173   NR, OS, NAP⁺:TM, PN

Mackay, C. & Ault, L. D. A systematic approach to individualizing nursing care. *Journal of Nursing Administration.* January 1977, 7(1):39–48.

A systematic plan can be used to move nursing care from a functional, task-oriented approach to individualized nursing care meeting the physical, psychological, and social needs of patient. The successful implementation of individualized nursing care depends on having: (1) staff with skills, (2) resource persons available, (3) built-in in-service and continuing education program, and (4) nonclinical staff to assume nonclinical duties. The need for these elements cannot be overemphasized or underestimated. If the plan is fully implemented, it will provide demonstrable evidence of individualized nursing care. (Authors' abstract)

174   PC, NAP:TM

MacKay, M. Organization of nursing services for geriatric patients. In Schneweiss, S. M. & Davis, S. W. (eds.) *Nursing Home Administration.* Baltimore: University Park Press, 1974.

Discussion of organization of nursing services in nursing homes. A team method of assignment is described. Patient characteristics and resulting needs for services are described. (JB)

175   NAP⁺:PN

Manthey, M. Primary nursing is alive and well in the hospital. *American Journal of Nursing.* January 1973, 73(1):83–87.

Description of the implementation of primary nursing on several units. (BK)

176   NAP⁺:PN

Manthey, M., Ciske, K., Rooutsom, P. & Harris, I. Primary nursing: A return to the concept of 'my nurse and my patient.' *Nursing Forum.* January 1971, 9(1):65–83.

Description of the implementation of primary nursing on a 23-bed medical unit. (BK)

177   PC, NR, OS, NAP:PN

Manthey, M. & Kramer, M. A dialogue on primary nursing. *Nursing Forum.* 1970, 9(4):356–379.

The format of this article is a critical dialogue in which the theoretical and historical framework of primary nursing are reviewed. Included are discussions on staffing implications, patient care assignments, auxiliary personnel assignment, and quality control. (JC)

178   OS*, NAP:TM, FN

Maresca, A. A. An examination of the relationship between selected organizational variables and the performance of staff nurses in a general hospital. (Unpublished master's thesis, Arizona State University, 1973.)

The purpose of this descriptive study was to identify the influence of the social structure of an acute hospital setting on the role performance of staff nurses. The problem under investigation was as follows: In what way does the availability of patient service departments and the types and numbers of nursing staff influence the distribution of nursing activities? Operationalization of the research problem was accomplished through the utilization of Levinson's conceptualization of role theory. Data for information on the role performance of staff nurses were obtained through a nursing activity study by utilizing the work sampling technique. Each observed nursing activity was categorized into one of the following areas: patient-centered, personnel-centered, unit-centered or other-centered. Results demonstrated an associative relationship between the role performance of the staff nurse and the social structure of the acute hospital setting. As the availability of patient service departments increased, the amount of patient-centered activities performed by staff nurses decreased significantly. Regardless of the percent of availability of patient service departments, the distribution of actual nursing activities remained constant. Relationships between the numbers and types of nursing personnel and nursing activity distributions were not examined. Analysis also revealed that nursing activity distributions varied significantly between the three shifts. The greatest distribution of administrative activities were performed on shift I. The greatest distribution of actual nursing activities were performed on shift II. The greatest distribution of clerical activities were performed on shift III. On all three shifts the most frequent skill activity performed by the staff nurse was administration. (JC)

179   NAP*:TM, PN

Marram, G. The comparative costs of operating a team and primary nursing unit. *Journal of Nursing Administration.* May 1976, 6(4):21–24.

Aware of the administrator's concern with cost effectiveness, the author implemented a six-month study of the comparative operating costs of a primary nursing unit and a team care unit. She found salary costs and overall costs to be lower in the primary unit. This report is adapted from much larger report: Marram. G. *Cost-Effectiveness of Primary and Team Nursing.* Wakefield, Mass: Contemporary Publishing Co., 1976. (CAL)

180   NAP, OS

Mauksch, H. O. The nurse: Coordinator of patient care. In Skipper, J. K. & Leonard, R. C. *Social Interaction and Patient Care.* Philadelphia: J. B. Lippincott Company, 1965.

The author discusses the organization of the patient care unit and the role of the nurse within it, for the purpose of organizing existing knowledge as a basis for objective study and experimentation. In organizing the patient care unit, the nursing force performs duties other than direct patient care, tasks which reflect the structuring of functions of the institution and which are shaped by the organizational pattern of the hospital. Functions of management and coordination are discussed and related to administrative responsibilities. (JB)

181   PC, NAP*

McCarthy, C. Incentive reimbursement as an impetus to cost containment. *Inquiry.* December 1975, 12(4)320–329.

Description of an experiment in which nurse clinician coordinators for health maintenance activities with high-risk patients worked in community and hospital settings to reduce hospital admissions and length of stay. A decrease in both hospital discharge rate and length of stay in the experimental group was greater than in the control group, and cost savings resulted. Medicare patients with chronic medical conditions participated. (JB)

182   PC, NR

McCartney, R. A., Cady, L. D. & McKee, B. Nurse staffing systems. *Hospitals.* November 16, 1970, 44:102–106.

This article describes a formula for determining the number of nursing staff hours required per patient per day. Four categories of patients were delineated according to the kinds of nursing care required. Quantitative ratios were determined for the amount of care required in each category. The relative percentage of each category occurring in the average total patient load was determined. Hours of nursing time then were distributed by patient category, by type of staff and by shift. (JC)

183   PC

McCormick, P. et al. Predicting nurse staffing. *Hospitals.* May 1, 1973, 47:68–79.

This study analyzes the staffing at the Washington Hospital Center (D.C.). By statistical analysis of work sampling data on medical and surgical units, plus continuous observational data taken on selected patients from this analysis, significant relationships emerge that, when integrated with organizational requirements, can aid in the improvement of nurse staffing. The following 13 variables were found to account for 75% of the variance in time for direct patient care activities: assist with mobility, nothing by mouth, assist with feeding, some assist with bathing, complete assist with bathing, use of bedpan, incontinent, patient observation, suction turn and position, bed scale weight, dressing and isolation. (JC)

184   PC, NAP

McFadden, E. & Kopf, R. Integrated staffing for a special care unit. *Supervisor Nurse.* May 1975, 6(5):26–32.

Description of organizational method used to solve staffing problems in a rooming-in, family-centered maternity unit and an intensive care nursery in one hospital. This nursery originally existed in close proximity to the maternity unit, but was organized, supervised, and staffed by the Department of Pediatrics and the Pediatric Nursing Service. This division of services resulted in fragmentation of care and poor communication between staffs and patients. In an attempt to alleviate the problem, an eight-bed Neonatal Unit was developed adjacent to the postpartum unit, and steps were taken to assure a constant source of prepared nurses to staff the special care unit. The authors conclude that initiation of this "integrated staffing" plan has prevented patient and staff anxiety, the "no prepared staff" crisis, the disruption of the interpersonal process, and the development of an "intellectual ghetto" (i.e., an abundance of nursing staff prepared in a narrow specialty field). (CAL)

185   NR, OS

McKenna, J. V. Final project report: The service manager system: nurse efficacy and cost. Available from University Microfilms International, Ann Arbor, Mich. *Abstracts of Hospital Management Studies,* No. NU1065.

A surgical unit and medical unit with unit management were compared to traditionally managed surgical unit and medical unit at Barnes Hospital, St. Louis, in a three-year study. The activities of unit personnel, patient care, and cost were compared. Charge nurses and team leaders on both medical and surgical units with unit management spent more time on nursing level activities than nurses on the traditionally managed unit. A new type of nursing supervisor "with minimal administrative functions and strong patient care responsibilities" was a factor in the development of the lay managed units. There was no significant difference in patient welfare (equated with rate of recovery) on the two differently managed units. Data on cost were inconclusive; nursing care could not be measured directly; and no significant differences were found in length of stay on the test units. It was found that service management did focus nursing activities on patient care; service personnel took over functions performed by nurses; and service management is equal to traditional management in providing for patient welfare. (Abstract adapted from Jelinek, Munson & Smith, *Service Unit Management,* p. 102. Battle Creek, Mich.: W. K. Kellogg Foundation, February 1971.)

186   PC*, NAP*

McKim, S. A study of the effect of the case assignment of a nurse upon the post-hospital separation anxiety behaviors of hospitalized toddlers. (Unpublished master's thesis, University of Rochester, New York, 1973.) Available from University Microfilms International, Ann Arbor, Mich. *Abstracts of Hospital Management Studies,* No. 11692NU.

This pilot study was done to determine if the presence and care by the same nurse for part of every day of a toddler's hospitalization would decrease separation anxiety as demonstrated by the child's behavior at home one week after discharge from the hospital. Case assignment/primary nurse assignment was the experimental variable, defined as assignment of a specific nurse to specific patients for the length of hospitalization, with primary responsibility for planning and implementing care for the patient and provision of all care while on duty. The control group assignment pattern was team nursing, with change in the care assignment almost every day. The dependent variable was separation anxiety, measured by behaviors in the areas of dependency, eating habits, and sleep patterns. Findings were that positive behaviors occurred more frequently in the experimental group than in the control, while negative behaviors occurred more frequently in the control group. Conclusions were that the experimental (case/primary) group children experienced less trauma from separation anxiety than the control (team) group. Several important variables were uncontrolled in this study, including time spent with children by their mothers in the hospital (other than the fact that none used rooming-in), and bias introduced by the investigator in the experimental situations and in data collection. (JB)

187   OS, NAP⁺:PN

Mealy, S., Kiener, M., Mann, J. & Simandl, G. Shared leadership—no head nurse! *Nursing Administration Quarterly.* Fall 1976, 1(1):81–93.

Description of patient care organization and unit coordination at Family Hospital, Milwaukee, Wis., on a medical unit. Staff nurses share leadership without head nurse or charge person; adaptation of primary nursing is the assignment pattern. (JB)

188   OS, NR, NAP

Medicus Systems Corporation. *A review and evaluation of nursing productivity. Vol. I and II. Conference Proceedings and Final Report.* Chicago: The Corporation, October 1975, January 1976.

Proceedings of a conference and final summary of the activities, findings, and recommendations of a project to review and evaluate previous efforts to measure and improve the productivity of nursing personnel. Activities reported include: investigation of various definitions of nursing productivity, development of a conceptual framework, literature search, evaluation of research on nursing productivity, presentation and refinement of the findings and recommendations at a national conference of leaders in the fields of nursing, administration, and education. Companion volume is *Vol. III. Literature and Research Review,* Chicago: The Corporation, November 1975. (JB)

189   OS

Mendelov, D. *A study of various organizational arrangements of the unit manager system.* Available from University Microfilms International, Ann Arbor, Mich. *Abstracts of Hospital Management Studies,* No. NU1184.

This study attempts to determine at what level of authority Unit Managers function most effectively in hospital nursing units. Questionnaires were sent to selected hospitals employing Unit Managers, conferences were held with representatives of active programs, and a pilot program was used for first-hand observa-

tion. The author concluded the Unit Manager would be a coequal of the charge nurse, but should be organizationally placed under administration rather than nursing. (From *Abstracts of Hospital Management Studies,* June 1970, VI: 145.) (JB)

190   NAP⁺:TM

Mercy Hospital. *A manual for team nursing.* Pittsburgh, Pa.: Catholic Hospital Association, 1968.

Guide to implementation of team nursing. Includes discussion of philosophy, roles, and mechanism involved in team nursing. Steps to "successful team nursing" are given. (JB)

191   NR*, NAP:TM

Mergan, F. C. *Personnel utilization in a flexible nursing unit organization.* (Unpublished doctoral dissertation, University of Iowa, Dept. of Industrial and Management Engineering,Iowa City, 1963.)

To determine the effect of flexible nursing unit organizational structure, two nursing units were subjected to an experimental treatment that involved concentrating ultimate authority over all unit personnel in the head nurse. This permitted a revision of unit organization structure, redefinition of unit team members' duties, and employment of a flexible staffing plan. Medical and surgical units, control and experimental, were studied. The change to authority concentration was expected to permit more effective response to patient needs, while expansion of the duties of auxiliary personnel was expected to improve utilization of all personnel because of decreasing specialization. Pertinent variables do not appear to be well defined or isolated. Work requirements for staffing prediction were based on direct care, measured according to the time spent in patients' rooms. Results were summarized as: (1) nursing personnel utilization improved, (2) nursing personnel work patterns changed, and (3) nursing personnel job satisfaction did not change. Apparent benefits are summarized. Interunit standardization of practices and procedures occurred. It is suggested that consolidation of authority permitted a natural progress of personnel development within the team. (Adapted from review by M. Aydelotte, *Nurse Staffing*

Methodology, p. 189–195, DHEW Pub. No. (NIH) 73–433, January 1973.)

192   PC*, NR*, OS*, NAP*

Miller, S. J. & Bryant, W. D. *A division of nursing labor: Experiments in staffing a municipal hospital.* Kansas City, Missouri: Community Studies, Inc., 1965.

Variables of personnel utilization are examined and nursing activity investigated in nursing situations which provided minimal levels of nursing hours per patient, levels of approx. 2.0 or less. Independent variables included staff mix variations, in-service training, personnel preparation, and degree of care required by patients. Dependent variables included omissions in nursing care activities and quality of care. Hypotheses tested and results were as follows: Staff mix—Rate of omissions in nursing care would be directly related to (1) type of staffing pattern employed (staff mix) (supported); (2) number of nursing care hours per patient (supported); (3) degree of care required by patients (not supported). In-service training— would result in (1) a more appropriate distribution of nursing activities according to ability (supported for RN-LPN-aide mix, in part for other mixes); (2) increase in quality of care (partly supported), and decrease in omissions in care (not supported). Personnel preparation— (1) activity profiles of atypical and typical personnel would differ (supported for RNs and aides); (2) atypical staff would demonstrate increase in quality of care (supported), and decrease in rate of omissions compared to typical staff (not supported). Conclusions as to critical variables in adequate staffing and implications for productivity and quality are given. (JB)

193   NR

Moore, M. A. The professional practice of nursing: The knowledge and how to use it. *Nursing Forum.* 1969, 8(4):361–371.

This author proposes that no differentiation that meets everyone's satisfaction can be found between the technical versus the professional nurse. She proposes that the problem be approached from a different angle. The author contends that it is not who performs a nursing activity or how it is performed that determines whether the performance in question is to be regarded as professional in nature. She contends that the professional-technical distinction should be based on the activity involved. The questions are: (1) Are there functions carried out by the nurse that can be carried out only by a nurse who has had some special content in her educational program? (2) Is this content such that it would be impossible for it to be assimilated in a short training program? (JC)

194   NR, OS

Moxley, P. A. *The clinical nurse specialist: a study of behaviors characteristic of professional autonomy.* (Unpublished doctoral dissertation, Columbia University, 1973.)

The purpose of this study was to describe those behaviors which the clinical nurse specialists demonstrate in the performance of their work role that are characteristic of the professionally autonomous person. The data were gathered by direct observation of the specialists as they functioned in their roles. The sample consisted of seven clinical specialists, all of whom held Master's degrees. The specialties represented by the sample were Medical-Surgical Nursing, Maternal-Child Nursing and Nurse Midwifery. The practice settings for the specialists were two large metropolitan medical centers (four specialists in one, three in the other). Each was observed for one week. Based on the results of a pilot study, four categories were developed for the purposes of classifying the observed behaviors. These categories were: Nurse-Patient Interactions, Nurse-Other Health Professionals Interactions, Nurse-Institution Interactions, and Nurse-Self. An operational definition was developed to delineate the dimensions of professionally autonomous behaviors. The behaviors within each category were analyzed using the definition, and were classified as autonomous, interdependent or dependent in nature. Generally, the data demonstrated that the clinical nurse specialists do exhibit behaviors characteristic of a professionally autonomous person. (From Author's abstract)

195   OS, NAP:PN

Mundinger, M. O. Primary nursing: Impact on the education department. *Nursing Administration Quarterly.* Winter 1977, 1(2):69–77.

This article is an overview of some issues which arise for the staff educator related to the implementation of primary nursing. These issues encompass education that facilitates role changes, skill preparation, and learning the nursing process model of problem solving for patients. (JC)

197   NR, PC

National League for Nursing. *Providing a climate for the utilization of nursing personnel.* New York: The League, 1975. Pub. No. 20–1566.

Papers presented at the joint program of the National League for Nursing and the American Hospital Association, November 1974 in New York City. Focus of the report is the nursing process, with special emphasis on the utilization and preparation of nurses. Impact of shorter lengths of stay and the increasingly acute nature of hospital treatment is discussed by Donaho. Relationships between the nursing process, the skill required to accomplish it, and educational preparation is discussed by Yura. Other papers present views on various types of preparation in nursing education. (JB)

198   PC, NR

The National League of Nursing Education, The Committee on Studies. *A study of the nursing service in fifty selected hospitals.* (Reprinted from the *Hospital Survey for New York,* 2(5):355–429.) New York: The United Hospital Fund of New York, 1937.

The purpose of this study of nursing service in 50 acute general hospitals was "to find out how well hospital patients are nursed in New York City." Thirty-one voluntary, one county, and 18 municipal hospitals were chosen. The number of bedside nursing hours provided patients in the four basic services—medical, surgical, obstetric, and pediatric—in these institutions was obtained. The hours of care cited included time given by graduate nurses, student nurses, attendants, orderlies, and ward helpers. The time provided was examined in terms of type of hospital, basic service, and shift. Assessment of other factors included: the ratio of supervisors and head nurses to patients, the ratio of supervisors and head nurses to bedside workers, the extent to which nonprofessional workers are employed for bedside care, and the balance between patient load and bedside workers in the different hospitals. Recommendations based on study findings included the following: suggested minimum number of hours of bedside service per patient in each 24-hour period, by type of service studied; the number and kinds of personnel needed and the numbers of hours of employment of those personnel needed for any hospital nursing service. Further study and research about the factors reviewed was strongly recommended. (From *Planning for Nursing Needs and Resources.* DHEW Pub. No. (NIH) 72–87, App. 2, p. 156, April 1972)

199   PC, NR

The National League of Nursing Education, Department of Studies. *A study of nursing service.* New York: The League, 1948.

This was a study of the nursing services in one children's hospital and 21 general hospitals in the New York City area reputed to be well managed and to be providing high quality nursing care. An intensive study was made of the nurse-patient ratios in these hospitals and the duties performed by nonprofessional nursing personnel trained on the job. In all of the hospitals except one, the general hours of nursing care actually given per patient were fewer than the hours needed. The average ratio was 3.5 hours of nursing care per patient per day, of which two-thirds was provided by registered nurses and one-third by nursing aides, practical nurses, and others. The study provided medians to be used as guides in determining the nursing needs of medical, surgical, obstetrical, and pediatric patients in general hospitals. Measures to improve the training, supervision, and utilization of nursing aides in hospitals were also recommended. (From *Planning for Nursing Needs and Resources.* DHEW Pub. No. (NIH) 72–87, App. 2, p. 156–7, April 1972)

200   NR, OS, NAP⁺:PN

Nehls, D., Hansen, V., Manthey, M. & Robertson, P. Planned change: A quest for nursing autonomy. *The Journal of Nursing Administration.* January-February 1974, 4(1):23–27.

Description of the implementation of primary nursing on a unit, with subsequent extension to other units; total reorganization of the nursing department from a hierarchical to decentralized authority is also described. (BK)

201 OS

Nellis, W. L. Unit managers cut patients' complaints 50 percent. *Hospital Topics.* June 1968, 46:42-45.

A report on the development of a unit-management program in Beth Israel Hospital, Boston. An improvement in the working relationship between employee groups was noted and 50 percent reduction in complaints of patients occurred. Costs of supplies decreased even though census increased. The unit manager reported to administration. (JB)

202 NR, NAP⁺:PN

Nenner, V. C., Curtis, E. M. & Eckhoff, C. M. Primary nursing. *Supervisor Nurse.* May 1977, 8(5):14-16.

Brief description of philosophy of primary nursing, its implementation at one particular hospital, and the outcomes in terms of patient, doctor, and nurse satisfaction. This article is unclear whether there is 24-hour responsibility assumed by one nurse, or only responsibility for the 8-hour shift she works. (CAL)

203 PC, OS, NR⁺, NAP:PN

Nield, M. Developing a projected nurse staffing program. *Supervisor Nurse.* July 1975, 6(7): 17-18, 20-24.

According to the author, "the objective of a nurse staffing program is to determine the number and kind of nursing personnel required to provide nursing care of a predetermined standard for a specific group of patients in a particular setting." In the fall of 1976 the Pima County General Hospital staff moved to a modern 221-bed facility known as Kino Community Hospital (KCH) in Tucson, Arizona. The consulting firm of Gordon A. Friesen International, Inc. recommended assigning 135 of the 221 beds to the adult medical-surgical service. This figure represented an increase of 41 beds over the number in the county hospital and necessitated the development of a new staffing program. This article discusses factors to be considered in predicting staffing needs in a new

facility. Selection of a nursing assignment pattern was considered an essential element of the staffing program; primary nursing was the suggested method. (CAL)

204 NAP⁺:TM

Nolan, M. Team nursing in the OR. *American Journal of Nursing.* 1974, 74:272-274.

The author describes her efforts, as charge nurse in an operating room area, to implement team nursing as a means to alleviate the problems of motivating, teaching, and supporting staff in a high-risk setting. The author found team nursing to be a positive force for the nurses and orderlies; however, the technicians, like the physicians, wanted the experienced nurses to circulate for them, rather than to function as team leaders. The concept did not become a permanent feature of the operating room, a result the author attributes to the lack of commitment to team approach and high turnover rate. (CAL)

205 OS

Norris, C. M. Direct access to the patient. *American Journal of Nursing.* May 1970, 70(5): 1006-1010.

This is a position paper regarding the value and necessity of patients having direct access to the professional nurse rather than having access only through physicians. Examples used provide primarily ambulatory care, and emphasize "nurse access to patients." Loeb Center is given as an example of a nursing hospital. (BK)

206 NAP⁺

The nurses' shift report, a CASH case study for maintaining continuity of inpatient care. *Hospital Forum.* June 1965, 8:11-13, 33.

Use of a Patient Care Plan form and tape recording of additional comments simplify shift report and allow ancillary personnel to begin work without delay. It also improves continuity of care by providing a written plan and documentation of care given, and can be related to staffing and allocation decisions. Relationships of various assignment patterns and continuity of care planning are discussed briefly. (JB)

207   NAP*:PN

O'Connell, E. M. & Grimm, S. A. The effect of consistent contact on the postoperative recovery of abdominal surgery patients. (Unpublished master's thesis, University of Michigan, 1976.)

The purpose of this study was to examine the effect of consistent versus inconsistent contact with patients, as one element of primary nursing, on patients' recovery from surgery. Seventy -nine surgical patients scheduled for either an abdominal hysterectomy or a cholecystectomy were randomly assigned to the experimental group or the control group. The experimental group received consistent daily contact for a five-day period with one of the nurse researchers. The subjects in the control group were seen in a random manner by one of the nurse researchers and never more than two consecutive days by the same researcher. The subjects in each group provided daily self-report recovery measures such as pain, medication used, time spent out of bed, etc. These were used to determine the patient's rate of recovery. On inhospital self-report recovery measures, there was a trend for the control group to report higher, or feeling better, than the experimental group on some of the questions. However, this trend never reached significance, and on the subjective measures the experimental and control groups were not significantly different in the pain medication they received. On posthospitalization self-report measures, the experimental group rated themselves as fully recovered from surgery six days sooner than the subjects in the control group. Interpretation of the findings of this study, as well as their implications for nursing, are discussed. (JB)

208   PC*

Overton, P., Hazlett, C. B. & Schneck, R. An empirical study of the technology of nursing subunits. *Administrative Science Quarterly.* June 1977, 22:203-219.

The purpose of this study was to describe and differentiate empirically the technology of seven types of nursing subunits (n=71) in hospitals. Technology was measured by a 34-item questionnaire given to a random sample of five nurses from each subunit (response rate 95.5 percent). Data analyses were performed on subunit scores. By factor analysis, three independent technological factors were identified, which were labelled uncertainty, instability, and variability. Significant differences (α=.05) between some of the types of subunits were shown in terms of these three factors. From the application of Q technique, three categories of nursing subunits were identified, which were interpreted in terms of their degree of indeterminacy of their technologies. (Author's abstract)

209   OS

Pablo, R. Y. Job satisfaction in a chronic care facility. *Dimensions in Health Services.* January 1976, 53(1):36–39.

The care of chronically ill persons in longterm facilities can lessen staff motivation and satisfaction, resulting in high turnover. Late in 1973, 86 staff members of an extended care and rehabilitation center for the chronically ill indicated their agreement or disagreement with 50 factors which may increase or decrease motivation and satisfaction of staff employed in an organizational system. Most (92 percent) respondents were female; 43 percent were nursing staff, 48 percent were nonnursing staff. Employees above the mean age of 34 years reported significantly lower interpersonal anxiety than the younger employees. The sense of accomplishment and importance was significantly higher for male employees. Nonnursing staff rates themselves lower on interpersonal anxiety and difficulties compared to the nursing staff. The esteem factor was higher for nursing staff. Respondents in administrative positions experienced less esteem conflict, anxiety, and rejection than those in nonadministrative positions. Increasing years of service correlated with a greater sense of accomplishment and importance. The overall response reflected relative satisfaction by the majority. Dissatisfaction among 35 percent on the esteem factor, however, was considered worthy of attention. Although salary, hours, and fringe benefits may initially attract an employee, response to sociopsychological needs of the individual influences retention and performance. Regular appraisal of the adequacy of external and internal rewards in a care facility can provide information for decreasing the anxiety of employees, improving self-esteem and security, and resolving problems which affect productivity and retention. (Abstract from *Nursing Research,* Jan.-Feb. 1977)

210 NR⁺, NAP:PN

Page, M. Primary nursing: Perceptions of a head nurse. *American Journal of Nursing.* August 1974, 74(8):1435–1438.

The author describes the head nurse's task on a primary nursing unit as consultant and developer. On the primary nursing unit, there is a head nurse, a secretary, and primary nurse; while the head nurse is available when nursing judgement is required, the secretary is responsible for the hourly administration of work on the unit. The head nurse also has primary patients and is also responsible for making assignments. Criteria for making assignments are the patient's needs, the nurse's skills, and nurse's needs. Nurses are on rotating shifts on this unit. (JC)

211 PC, NR, OS, NAP:TM

Palisin, H. E. Nursing care plans are a snare and a delusion. *American Journal of Nursing.* 1971, 71(1):63–66.

The value of nursing care plans for patients is questioned by the author. The limitations of this communication method in the hospital work setting are discussed. Palisin asserts that nursing care plans may have some value for patients who are acutely ill and cannot communicate, but proliferation of such a tool for all patients not only complicates the communication process but interferes with individualized care. (From *Planning for Nursing Needs and Resources,* DHEW Publication No. (NIH) 72-87, p. 162, April 1972.)

212 PC, NR

Pardee, G. Classifying patients to predict staff requirements. *American Journal of Nursing.* March 1968, 68(3):517–520.

Description of the development of a patient classification system at the University Hospital in Seattle, Washington. Patients were classified according to their nursing needs in order to predict staffing requirements. (BK)

213 NAP

Passos, J. Y. Accountability: Myth or mandate. In Nursing Digest (ed.), *Focus on Professional Issues.* Wakefield, Mass.: Contemporary Publishing, 1975.

Accountability is defined as answering to someone for something that one has done (Peplau). Nurses in agencies as employees are accountable to the employer and/or physician. Only private practitioners are accountable directly to the recipient of nursing care. Professional norms indicate that professionals should be judged by peers and responsible to recipients; thus peer review and strategies for assigning or using nurses which require the nurse to be responsible to the recipient for services provided are necessary for truly professional accountability to occur. In addition, continuity in the nursing process (of personnel as well as plan), standards of practice, improved documentation of care, and evaluation of both process and outcome of care and peer evaluation and cost analysis are needed. (JB)

214 OS, NAP⁺:FN, TPC?

Pembrey, S. From work routine to patient assignment: An experiment in ward organization. *Nursing Times.* November 6, 1975, 71(45):1768–1772.

This article discusses the problems encountered in implementing patient assignment patterns instead of task assignment patterns. (JC)

215 PC, NR, NAP

Perrow, C. A framework for the comparative analysis of organizations. In Maurer, J. G. (ed.), *Readings in Organization Theory: Open-System Approaches,* pp. 106–124. New York: Random House, 1971.

This distinctive paper presents a perspective on organizations for use as a basis for comparative analysis and to facilitate the selective use of existing theories of organizational behavior. Four characteristics of this perspective are described: (1) Technology is considered the defining characteristic of organizations. The discussion of technology includes its relevance to the organizational structure, the nature of the work in terms of exceptions encountered, and search processes used. (2) Technology is generally treated as an independent variable and structure as the dependent variable. Goals are conceived as dependent variables, at least in part. (3) The perspective attempts to conceptualize the organization as a whole. (4) The perspective holds that technology is a better basis for comparing organizations than other existing schemas. This perspective has much to offer as a basic framework for conceptualizing the organization and structure of nursing units. (JB)

216   NR, OS, NAP⁺:TM

Peterson, G. G. *Working with others for patient care.* 2nd edition. Dubuque, Iowa: William C. Brown Company, 1973.

A textbook on team leading and hospital organization for persons new to the principles of or interested in implementing team nursing. Extensive citation of principles useful in implementing team functioning, along with description of roles within the team, the health team, and the hospital system are included. The author espouses the view that the effectiveness of team nursing is the result of close working relationships, respect for various roles, better utilization of personnel, and greater supervision. The core element is the team conference, with the nursing care plan a valuable adjunct. Composition of the team is less important than the basic philosophy. (JB)

217   NAP⁺:TM

Phillips, E. C. A group approach to nursing service. *Nursing Outlook.* August 1965, 13(8): 46–49.

Report of the implementation of team nursing at the visiting nurse service of Rochester and Monroe County, New York. (CAL)

218   NAP⁺:PN

Pisani, S. H. Primary nursing—aftermath of change. *Nursing Administration Quarterly.* Winter 1977, 1(2):107–113.

This article is an account of: (1) the ways in which the change to primary nursing affected individual staff members and their interaction on the unit, (2) the reasons these reactions occurred, and (3) the process used in addressing the resulting problems. (JC)

219   PC, NAP⁺:CS

Prerequisite for nurse-physician collaboration: nursing autonomy. *Nursing Administration Quarterly.* Fall 1976, 1(1):49–50. (See also #154)

Panel presentation and audience interaction in program sponsored by National Joint Practice Commission at the ANA Convention, Atlantic City, June 1976. One of panel participants, Karren Kowalski, assistant professor at the School of Nursing, University of Colorado, Denver and clinical specialist in obstetrics and gynecological nursing, describes a primary care system for both outpatient and inpatient obstetrical nursing care. Labor and delivery nurses follow a caseload of patients all the way through antepartum period in the clinic, give care in labor and delivery, and make rounds in postpartum unit. Both nurses and patients have increased satisfaction. (JB)

220   NR, OS, NAP

Price, E. M. *Staffing for patient care.* New York: Springer Publishing Company, Inc., 1970.

Part I of this report is a guide for introducing cyclical staffing. Part II of this report describes the study. Cyclical staffing was introduced as the experimental variable in five hospitals. Intervening and dependent variables related to staffing were studied. Quality of care was not assessed. Cyclical staffing was indicated as most beneficial to hospital personnel. (JB)

221   PC, NR

Price, E. M. Staffing: The most basic nursing service problem. *Supervisor Nurse.* July 1975, 6(7):26-31. (See also #220)

The author is a "well known nurse consultant and author, best known for her research on staffing patterns." This article reviews methods which can be utilized by hospitals to "improve their staffing so that the level of staffing directly relates to the needs of the patients." The methods presented were developed by a research group directed by the author in Minneapolis-St. Paul hospitals, and are described in her book, *Staffing for Patient Care* (Springer) and are summarized in an *American Journal of Nursing* article in October, 1970. (CAL)

222   OS, NAP⁺:TPC

Race, G. A. T.P.C., a plan with R.N.'s at the center. *RN*. April 1974, 37(4):34–35.

Brief, general description, from doctor's viewpoint, of primary nursing on a medical unit. The NAP presented is labelled TPC (total patient care) and is described as a "nurse-centered plan." The following statements are some of the highlights of this article: RNs on the day shift are usually responsible for 4–5 patients each. The care they give includes serving the breakfast and lunch, giving the baths, doing bed checks, and making rounds with the doctors. Those on the 3 P.M.–11 P.M. shift may care for as many as 8 patients each, since only one meal is served, and other routine work is generally lighter. Those on the night shift may care for 11–12 patients each. Instead of using the nurses' station as her/his headquarters, the TPC nurse does her/his charting and gets meds and other supplies from the nurse-server, a flat-topped, desk-like cabinet, conveniently located between the rooms of her patient. Putting the nurse closer to the patient has meant that other services in the hospital have had to assume more responsibilities. With the nurse as the central figure, most of the services now seem more aware of their basic purpose: to help provide expert, healing care and make the patient's stay as comfortable as possible. In a recent unsigned questionnaire, 99 percent of the medical floor nurses gave their approval to TPC; several departments (in the hospital) have expressed their approval. TPC has made possible the grouping of medical patients with similar conditions in the same or adjoining rooms so that nurses with particular interests and skills can utilize them more effectively. From the doctor's viewpoint—and probably the nurse's—the most encouraging aspect is that the TPC nurse gets to spend much more time with patients. (CAL)

223   NR*

Reichow, R. W. & Scott, R. E. Study compares graduates of two-, three-, and four-year programs. *Hospitals*. July 16, 1976, 50(14):95–100.

Administrators and directors of nursing services were asked to rank new graduates of diploma, associate degree, and baccalaureate programs on ten characteristics. The survey was done in 166 hospitals and 34 skilled nursing homes in Kansas. Rankings are compared for hospitals with more than 100 beds, and hospitals with less than 100 beds; descriptive data from the nursing homes are described. The data showed that larger institutions have a higher regard for baccalaureate graduates than do the smaller ones, although both have a high opinion of diploma nurses. Responses indicated slightly higher baccalaureate ranking on leadership criteria. In areas of technical nursing, diploma nurses were favored regardless of institutional size. The associate degree nurses failed to demonstrate any areas of strength in comparison to the other graduates. Additional questionnaire items indicate little differences in starting salaries in most institutions, advancement criteria not based on educational preparation, and that eventually graduates of all three programs become equal in their ability to perform in the hospital setting within six months to two years. The criteria and discussion primarily reflect the values and concerns of institutions and employers of nursing personel. (JB)

224   OS, NAP⁺:TM

Registered Nurses' Association of Ontario. *Report, RNAO project for team nursing development*. Ontario: The Association, Jan. 1, 1971 to March 31, 1972.

Report of the second phase of a project to implement team nursing throughout the province of Ontario, beginning in 24 agencies/schools and later extending to other agencies. A report of the first 15 months was published in December, 1970. A supplemental report describing the plan of extension to other agencies was published in August, 1972. This skill development project evolved in three phases: (1) Conference for Directors of Nursing (June, 1968), (2) Initial Development of Team Nursing (September, 1969–March, 1972), (3) Development of Team Nursing in New Agencies (began September, 1972). Core group in each agency, composed of senior administrative personnel, appeared important to success. Evaluation was done by questionnaires; focus was on role performance of supervisor, head nurse, and team leaders, and the frequency of use of team leading tools. Progress in implementing team nursing required careful planning, adequate time for changes to be accepted, and consistent support both within and without the agency. Much helpful material on implementation; evaluation appeared rather subjective. (JB)

225   PC, NAP⁺

Riley, M. & Moses, J. A., Jr. Coordinated care: Making it a reality. *Journal of Nursing Administration*. April 1977, 7(4):21–25.

Describes development of a coordinated care program in which a core team works in cooperation with the patient's primary physician to provide interdisciplinary coordination and continuity of care for patients disabled by neurological catastrophe. The team, in addition to the physician and nurses caring for the patient, included a neurologist, physiatrist, nurse coordinator, public health nurse, and social worker. The nurse coordinator was a new position created for the program. The program included an automatic referral system, delineation of progressive phases of treatment, and protocols specifying basic medical and nursing procedures for all patients in the program. (JB)

226   PC, NAP⁺:CS

Rising, S. S. A consumer-oriented nurse-midwifery service. *Nursing Clinics of North America*. June 1975, 10(2):251–262.

Describes implementation of the Nurse-Midwifery Service; nurse-midwife assumes responsibility for normal prenatal, labor, delivery, and postpartum management, thus maintaining continuity of care. (JB)

227   PC, OS, NR

Robinson, A. M. Overview: New challenge for with-it nurses. *RN*. Jan. 1972, 35(1):31–39; The RN: Without her, no ICUs. *RN*. March 1972, 35(3):46–51; The nurse/doctor game (new style): Professional conflict in the ICU/CCU. *RN*. May 1972, 35(5):40–45, 101; Ongoing inservice programs are a must. *RN*. July 1972, 35(7):50–56; Intensive care today—and tomorrow: A summing-up. *RN*. September 1972, 35(9):56–60. (Available in book form ($3.00/copy) from ICU Survey Book, Box 48, c/o *RN* magazine, Oradell, N.J. 07649.)

Report of results of *RN* magazine's ICU 1972 survey in which valid replies to a 19-item questionnaire were received from 1,111 hospitals, all of which have 100 beds or more. The editors believe this to be the pioneer study of the relatively new professional field of ICU/CCU nursing. The questions elicited data on types of facilities and where they are located; numbers of beds in each facility; number and types of personnel; physician availability in ICU/CCU; description of "typical" RN who works in an ICU/CCU; preparation, in-service, orientation, and on the job training for nurses in ICU/CCU; types of tasks each level of personnel performs; salaries; nurse-doctor relations; lines of authority; use of "float" personnel; future trends. Questionnaires were filled out by the directors of nursing. (CAL)

228   NAP⁺:PN

Robinson, A. M. Primary-care nursing at two teaching hospitals. *RN*. April 1974, 37(4):31–34.

Brief general description of implementation, elements, and philosophy of primary nursing at the University of Minnesota (program started in 1958) and University of Rochester's Strong Memorial Hospital (program started in 1972). This NAP apparently allows for individualization of patient care based on the patient's needs and desires. Staff participation is voluntary; although no data are available, it is generally felt that the nurses and patients experience higher satisfaction with care under primary nursing. Another finding at the University of Minnesota is that the primary nurse spends about 70 percent of her or his time giving direct patient care. Comprehensive care and continuity of care are achieved through the combination of primary nurses, associate nurses, and other staff. Another finding of the Minnesota study is that not all nurses are prepared for nor want to assume the responsibility of primary care. (CAL)

229   PC, NR, NAP⁺:PN

Romero, M. & Lewis, G. Patient and staff perceptions as a basis for change. *Nursing Clinics of North America*. June 1977, 12(2): 197–203. (See also #086)

Lack of sufficient numbers and type of qualified nursing personnel necessitated the use of a team-functional organization of nursing care delivery on this medical unit. This resulted in fragmented, poor quality care, further resulting in both staff and patient dissatisfaction. In an attempt to alleviate this situation, the unit described in this article volunteered to be one of the four units attempting a new approach to nursing care delivery: modular-primary. This type of organization has resulted in higher quality of care and increased satisfaction. (JB)

230   OS, NAP:PN

Rotkovich, R. The role of the director of nursing in creating an environment for the practice of nursing. *Journal of the New York State Nurses' Association,* July 1973, 4(1):20-25.

Major areas affecting the role of director of nurses, as identified in this article, include: (1) the director's self-perception and quest for additional knowledge/education to facilitate effective leadership, (2) switching leadership styles as needed to be effective, (3) support for additional education for staff nurses, and (4) place in the organizational structure. The author sees the role of director of nurses as crucial, but her/his influence is dependent on self-appreciation of her or his own importance and the firmness used to defend her or his principles and standards of patient care. (JB)

231   NR, NAP:PN

Rotkovitch, R. The AD nurse: A nursing service perspective. *Nursing Outlook.* April 1976, 24(4):234-236.

This somewhat chatty article presents issues related to the skills the AD graduate is capable of as a staff nurse from the nursing service administrator's point of view, which are then contrasted to the views voiced by educators. Relevant comments are addressed to the AD graduate and the field of primary nursing. (JC)

232   PC, NR[+], NAP:TM

Ryan, T., Barker, B. L. & Marciante, F. A. A system for determining appropriate nurse staffing. *Journal of Nursing Administration.* June 1975, 5(5):30-38.

The staffing system whose implementation is discussed in this paper includes an assessment of the patients' nursing needs based on Kakosh's categories of nursing care needs, flexibility in assigning staff so that personnel with appropriate knowledge and skills are used for selected nursing functions, and current data which allow immediate compensation for under-or overstaffing. Team nursing was the assignment pattern in effect. (JB)

233   PC*, NR*, NAP:TM

Safford, B. J. & Schlotfeldt, R. M. Nursing service staffing and quality of nursing care. *Nursing Research.* Summer 1960, 9(3):149-154.

An experimental study was conducted to test the hypothesis that quality of nursing care would decrease as the number of patients assigned to nurses increased. An instrument was designed to assess quality of nursing care as defined by nursing personnel, physicians, hospital administrators, and patients in one institution. The quality of nursing care provided medical and surgical patients was assessed by both patients and personnel when assignments of 13, 16, and 19 patients were made to nursing teams, each composed of one registered nurse and two practical nurses. Findings generally supported the hypothesis. Responses from all personnel revealed assessment of decreased quality as assignments increased. Patients however showed little change in their evaluation of care under the three staffing patterns. Nurses and physicians reported marked decreases in quality as assignments increased. The category physical care showed a greater decrease in quality than did all other categories. Of the five categories of nursing care identified as essential, teaching and preparation for home care was consistently evaluated by all respondents to be less well accomplished than physical care, emotional care, nurse-physician relationships, and administration. Little difference was demonstrated between quality of care provided medical versus surgical patients under each of the three staffing patterns. The study concludes that workload of nursing personnel definitely relates to quality of care provided patients. (JB)

234   NAP*:TM

Schmieding, N. J. & Roberts, M. L. The effects of team nursing in staff-patient interaction. *Perspectives in Psychiatric Care.* 1967, 5(4):182-188.

This study was undertaken to accumulate

evidence which might indicate whether team nursing was effective in a psychiatric inpatient situation. The dependent variable was staff-patient interactions; there were no measurements of patient improvement. The greatest change occurred in the number and location of RN interactions with patients; the number of interactions and the number of minutes of interactions increased during team nursing, with fewer interactions taking place in the nursing office. The most substantial change in type of interaction was in the emotional-supportive category, which increased during team nursing. (JC)

235   PC*

Seay, A. B. & Wright, P. Nursing staffing decisions. Available from University Microfilms International, Ann Arbor, Mich. *Abstracts of Hospital Management Studies,* No. 14236NU.

This study evaluated and compared two nurse staffing schemes using data collected on two medical and two surgical units at Oakwood Hospital, Dearborn, Michigan, during an 18-day period from January 7 to January 24, 1975. The two schemes used were a patient classification scheme of four patient care categories and the PETO method developed for Oakwood Hospital which utilized a list of 34 nursing activities, each with a weighted average applied. Weights were determined by the degree of severity related to performance of the task. Daily census data did not vary significantly on study units, occupancy never falling below 85 percent and very often at 100 percent. Findings indicate patient classification scheme was a much simpler and faster method to apply. The PETO method of developing weights for nursing activities and relating this to number of staff needed to care for patients was found to be a lengthy process. Study found nursing care needs of medical unit remained high all week, including the weekend, whereas surgical unit's needs decreased on the weekend. However, both methods tended to staff surgical units with more personnel per required needs than they staffed medical units per required needs. Staffing tended to decrease on weekends in all units despite the fact that other units do not vary in their needs as surgical units do. Study concluded that the classification scheme could be adopted for use at Oakwood Hospital if data for

a larger sample are collected to verify trends and patterns of patient care needs. (Abstracted in *Abstracts of Hospital Management Studies,* June 1976, 12: 220.)

236   NR

Sheahan, D. The game of the name: Nurse professional and nurse technician. *Nursing Outlook.* July 1972, 20(7):440-444.

This article is a statement of opinion that focuses on the following issues: (1) There are several levels of nursing education but only one level of nursing practice. (2) Decision-making power is inherent in professional practice. (3) The professional practice of nursing calls for a new type of nurse-patient relationship and a new type of nursing authority. Author emphasizes that it is the physician's orders and his or her role expectations of nurses which are the chief determinants of the nurse's actions in hospital settings. There is a role and room in hospitals for the nursing administrator, the educator, the nurse researcher, and the nurse technician. But the professional nurse who practices in a hospital setting will probably function below her professional capacity, at a semiprofessional or technical level. Author contends that the clinical nursing specialist with advanced preparation has not been conspicuously successful in realizing the goals of clinical specialization. Two reasons are cited for this: (1) The general level of hospital nursing is on a technical level. (2) Clinical specialists lack decision-making power in most hospitals. (JC)

237   NR, NAP

Simmons, L. and Henderson, V. *Nursing research—a survey and assessment.* New York: Appleton-Century-Crofts, 1964.

This survey report and guide to nursing studies describes the beginnings of nursing research, the directions it has taken, and the forces which have impeded or promoted its development. A field survey of opinion in 27 states and a summary of problems identified by nurses, physicians, hospital administrators, educators, and others is reported. A system for classifying nursing studies is presented. The major part of the report is devoted to a review and assessment of research in selected occupational areas and nursing care, including surveys of nursing resources; image, role, and function studies including hospital ward studies; studies in clinical specialties and evaluative research. (Adapted from preface)

238   PC, OS, NAP*:CS, or PN

Sjoberg, K., Bicknell, P., Heieren, E. L. & Wilson, A. C. *Nursing study—phase III—the assessment of unit assignment in a multiward setting.* Saskatoon, Saskatchewan, University of Saskatchewan, August 1971. (See also #239)

Discussion of the implementation and results of the "unit assignment system" developed during phase II of this five-year study. On admission and on each day of their stay, patients are classified as requiring intense, above average, average, or minimal care. They are placed in the unit best equipped and staffed to meet their needs. A unit is defined as "that number of patients who can be cared for by a registered nurse given adequate nursing assistance and supply services." Units are defined by day shift workload and are merged or combined during evening and night shifts. The typical assignment then is a nurse and her assistant to a group of patients, the number of patients depending on their classification. Weekly assignments are prepared by the head nurse. Implementation and results, including comparison with team nursing on the same units, in terms of achievement of standards, changes in attitudes, and costs, are described. (JC)

239   PC, OS, NAP+:CS or PN

Sjoberg, K. B., Heieren, E. L. & Jackson, M.R. Unit assignment: A patient-centered system. *Nursing Clinics of North America.* June 1971, 6(6):333–342. (See also #238)

Description of the unit assignment system, based on patient classification, designed to provide effective personalized patient care closely matched to patients' needs. In unit assignment, ward structure is decentralized and divided into units of care, classified as the number of patients that can be effectively cared for by an RN given adequate nursing assistance and supplies. Emphasis is given to keeping like categories of patients together in a unit in order to predict and equalize the workload. The head nurse role is discussed as well as other organizational support systems necessary. Evaluation

suggests that unit assignment leads to improved patient care, improved utilization of nurses, continuity, and job satisfaction. (BK)

240   NAP+:PN

Smith, C. C. Primary nursing care—a substantive nursing care delivery system. *Nursing Administration Quarterly.* Winter 1977, 1(2):1–8.

This article enthusiastically identifies primary nursing as the "keystone to the rebirth of our hospital." Author cites the following topics: outcomes of primary nursing, key objectives, substantive factors which emerge as primary nursing is implemented, and organizational elements of primary nursing. (JC)

241   OS, NAP:PN

Sobczak, C. L. Pharmacy and primary nursing: Potential for conflict and cooperation. *Nursing Administration Quarterly.* Winter 1977, 1(2):89–96.

This article describes a conflict between two functionally interdependent departments—nursing and pharmacy—during the implementation of primary nursing. The change went from unit dose and team nursing to unit dose and primary nursing. Unfortunately, resulting modifications in the unit dose system are not described. (JC)

242   OS

Sperlbaum, A. *Bibliography of service unit management.* Available from University Microfilms International, Ann Arbor, Mich. *Abstracts of Hospital Management Studies,* No. NU1222. (See also #140)

"This annotated bibliography covers fifty-eight journal articles, theses and project reports which deal with experiences in nursing unit management." The period covered is 1952 to 1968. The following areas are covered in each annotation: (1) the job description of the unit manager, (2) the objectives to be attained, and (3) the experience each individual hospital had in implementing unit management. (Abstract from *Planning for Nursing Needs and Resources.* DHEW Pub. No. (NIH) 72-87, p. 161, April 1972)

243   PC

State University of New York at Buffalo, Faculty of Health Sciences, School of Nursing. *Development of computer manageable assessment forms which will provide patient care information for making nursing decisions.* Buffalo: State University of New York, February 1970.

This volume describes the planning, development, and qualitative evaluation of the application of nursing data forms to a computer-implemented hospital information system. Authors concluded that if data are available in a definite format—on a form—they are immediately more effectively applicable to a computer-implemented system than if they are unstructured. Thus, the nursing data forms in question are indeed applicable to a computer data processing system. Benefits of structured forms are described. (JC)

244   OS

Stevens, B. J. Analysis of trends in nursing care management. *Journal of Nursing Administration.* Nov.-Dec. 1972, 2(6):12–17.

Insightful article contrasting two distinct approaches to nursing measurement: the task analysis time study method and the nursing quality control approach. The focus is on developing a quality control system, and the necessary components of a quality control system are identified. Different types of standards are also identified and compared. (JB)

245

Stevens, B. J. Effecting change. *Journal of Nursing Administration.* February 1975, 5(2): 23–26.

Effecting change is an integral part of the nurse executive's role. Reasons for resistance to change are examined and stages in acceptance of change are given. Some of the nurse executive's resources for implementing change are identified and discussed. Factors of attitudinal and behavioral change are considered. The article is a chapter in the author's book, *The Nurse as Executive,* published by Contemporary Publishing, Inc., Wakefield, Massachusetts. (JB)

246   OS, NAP

Steward, D. Y. Nursing organization—Circa 1969. *The Canadian Nurse.* February 1969, 65(2):59–61.

This article describes an organizational pattern of nursing service in keeping with current needs to relieve nurses of nonnursing functions. Traditional organization is supplanted by changes in the roles and functions of key persons responsible for nursing administration in a hospital and by the decentralization of authority from the director of nursing to other nursing staff. The plan provides for a nursing administrator on each floor; a nursing coordinator, who is a clinical specialist, for each 30-bed unit; and floor managers responsible to hospital administration. (From *Planning for Nursing Needs and Resources,* DHEW Pub. No. (NIH) 72–87, p. 161, April 1972)

247   OS

Stryker, R. How does nursing home administration differ from hospital administration? *Journal of Nursing Administration.* May 1975, 5(4):16–17.

Nursing home care must begin with a different orientation than hospital care, because it is based on psychosocial rather than medical needs of patients.

248   OS, NAP:PN

Swanson, K. T. Primary nursing care as a management tool. *Nursing Administration Quarterly.* Winter 1977, 1(2):6–7.

This article describes how primary nursing affected a hospital that had a poor community reputation and was unable to recruit physicians. Primary nursing was implemented in order to recruit physicians and their patients to this hospital. (JC)

249   NAP*:TM

Swearingen, L. L. *An evaluation of an experimental reorganization of the nursing care delivery system.* Available from University Microfilms International, Ann Arbor, Mich. *Abstracts of Hospital Management Studies,* No. NU2007.

An effort to measure the impact of a revised job assignment for RNs and LPNs which instructed them to work as a two-nurse team and to avoid all duties which were not patient-related or clinical nursing. Although several different measures were undertaken, aimed at nurse satisfaction, patient satisfaction, and quality of care, the experimental conditions were severely limited by factors beyond the author's control. Sample sizes were very small and most measures showed no significant change. (From *Abstracts of Hospital Management Studies,* 1968, 4:165.)

250   PC, OS, NR, NAP⁺:TM

Thomas, L. A. Predicting change in nursing values. In Nursing Digest (ed.), *Focus on the Work Environment,* p. 126-134, Wakefield, Mass.: Contemporary Publishing, c. 1975.

Describes development of a program for appraising nursing competence at varying levels of expertise and experience, based on the Statement of Standards for Nursing Practice developed by the California Nurses Association. These standards incorporate the use of a patient acuity system in assessing patients' needs for nursing care and also set up essential protocols for the assignment of nurses to patients (Standards I and II). Ongoing evaluation of care and assignments is also included (Standard III). The standards are interpreted as criteria for planning, administering, and evaluating nursing care; and classifications of nurses according to their abilities to meet the standards were developed. Using these criteria, a Nurse Board of Review was formed to evaluate practice and promote nurses. This system was developed to replace a general employee appraisal form which was unrelated to professional practice. (JB)

251   PC*

Thompson, J. D., et al. Age a factor in amount of nursing care given, AHA study shows. *Hospitals.* March 1, 1968, 42(2):33-38.

A study of 55 general hospitals in nine areas of the United States, reports the effect of patient age, 65 or older, on the amount of nursing care received. On all shifts, within all subgroupings of hospitals and units, patients 65 and older received significantly more hours of care per patient than those younger than 65. The extra care ranged from 36 to 55 minutes per patient per day, or between 14 percent to 22 percent more hours of nursing care per patient than for adult patients under 65. The amount of this difference was greater in smaller hospitals, non-university affiliated hospitals, hospitals without student nurses, and hospitals with a low degree of effort specialization. There was no difference between medical and surgical units. (JB)

252   OS

Tobin, H. Quality staff development: A must for change and survival. *Journal of Nursing Administration.* May 1976, 6(4):39-42.

Notes growing acknowledgment in nursing that provision for continued education is a necessity for maintaining quality health care. Discusses how nursing administrators can effectively implement a program for continued education that will enable a staff to provide the highest quality of nursing service. This article is based on Standard IX of ANA's Standards for Nursing Services, 1973. (JB)

253   PC*

Trivedi, V. M., & Hancock, W. M. Measurement of nursing workload using head nurses' perceptions. *Nursing Research.* Sept.-Oct. 1975, 24(5): 371-376.

This study attempted to measure levels of need based on the perceptions of head nurses. A methodology for measuring and predicting workload on nursing units utilized perceptions of head nurses as measured by a specially designed questionnaire. Results indicated that head nurses' perceptions of need on nursing units were predominantly influenced by unit census and available staff on the unit. Other patient-load affecting variables, such as patient classification, number of new admissions, or postoperative patients, did not play a major role in shaping head nurses' perceptions. Eight variables were selected as candidates for establishing a relationship with severity of need: (1) nursing hours available for a shift, (2) unit census, (3) patient classification (number of type I, II, III, IV patients), (4) number of new admissions during a shift, (5) number of transfers out, in or within the unit, (6) number of discharges during shift, (7) number of 48-hour postop patients, and (8) number of "specialized" nursing procedures performed on shift. (JC)

254   OS*

Underwood, C. B. *Comparison of nursing activities before and after implementation of the patient unit management program.* Available from University Microfilms International, Ann Arbor, Mich. *Abstracts of Hospital Management Studies,* No. NU1103.

Study compared the proportion of time nurses spent in nonnursing activities before a patient-unit manager program began and afterwards, on a 49-bed surgical subspecialty unit for medically indigent patients at University of Alabama Hospital. Data from a work-sampling study of the unit in 1963, before introduction of Patient Unit Management, were compared to a 1966 study of the same unit with a patient unit manager. Study found total patient care activities, direct and indirect, increased from 40.5 percent in 1963 to 59.2 percent in 1966. Direct patient care showed greatest amount of increase. In addition, there was a 65.9 percent decrease shown in unit management activities performed by nursing personel. Comparisons by day of week, by hour, and by worker classification also demonstrate an increase in total and direct patient care and a decrease in unit management activities. Copies of obervation sheets used and statistical data from the study are included in the appendix. (From *Abstracts of Hospital Management Studies,* 1968, 4:161.)

255   NAP, NR

United States Department of Health, Education, and Welfare, Division of Nursing. *Planning for nursing needs and resources.* DHEW Pub. No. (NIH) 72–87, April 1972.

Presents basic guidelines and elements essential for effective planning for nursing, addressed primarily to the conduct of broad in-depth planning for all fields of nursing service, education, and for all types of nursing personnel within designated geographic areas. Appendix includes annotated bibliographies on survey and study reports, background material, and tools for planning. (JB)

256   NR, NAP:PN, TM, FN

University of Minnesota, Dept. of Conferences and Institutes. *Papers presented at the primary nursing institute.* Minneapolis: University of Minnesota, June 1971.

This booklet contains a compilation of addresses presented at a conference on primary nursing. All the articles are general knowledge based, as opposed to empirical studies. Papers address the history of assignment patterns, roles, educational preparation, clinical competence issues, and relations with other disciplines. (JC)

259   NAP⁺:CS

Waite, P. Specialty nursing teams in a small hospital. *RN*. February 1974, 37(2):34–35, 62, 64.

The author, who is director of nursing at the hospital, briefly describes the implementation of a program designed to increase the quality of nursing care through specialization. Inspired by the success of their 4-bed CCU, the hospital decided to expand the organizational and educaional framework of the CCU team to provide specialty teams in four other clinical areas: cancer, diabetes, respiratory disease, and stroke and rehabilitation. As an outgrowth of the specialty-team program, a committee for general patient care was added which helps with staff orientation and in-service education. Although no evaluation criteria are presented, the author states that "there are many evidences that our total program has helped increase the quality of nursing care generally as well as in the specialties." (CAL)

260   OS

Walker, V. H. *Nursing and ritualistic practice.* New York: The Macmillan Company, 1967. (See also #261)

A discussion based on results of several formal studies conducted by the author and also on her personal experiences. The formal studies were conducted to ascertain the extent of "ritualism" in a variety of duties which nurses perform. It was felt that some tasks were dysfunctional according to the achievement of the stated goal but served a ritualistic function for the performer. Tasks felt to be possibly ritualistic practices for the nurses were the taking of temperature, pulse, and respiration, writing of nurses' notes, use of the special report, and preparing and communicating the shift report. Each of these activities was studied; the specifics for obtaining the information varied for each study. Also included are the results observed in a ward when a ward manager was assigned to many administrative tasks normally relegated to the nursing staff. There is also discussion of the effect of the increasing bureaucratization of the hospital resulting in multiple subordination of the nurse, and increased absence of the doctor from the ward, thereby creating a lack of communication in the nurse-doctor relationship. (LJ) (From *Abstracts of Hospital Management Studies,* 1968, 4:164.)

261   OS*, NAP:TM

Walker, V., Hawkins, J. L. & Selmanoff, E. D. *Ritualism in nursing and its effects on patient care.* Final Research Report for USPHS, 1961–1964. (See also #260)

The major hypothesis which guided this research project was: Ritualistic procedures are a major factor in current nursing practice, and their use is a deterrent to the development of professional nursing judgement. The strategy used was to empirically establish the effect of some nursing behavior and then to infer its contribution (positively or negatively) to patient welfare. Ritualistic behavior was operationally defined as repetitive acts which are judged by nursing service administrators to be dysfunctional (unnecessary, useless, undesirable) in achieving adequate patient care and are believed to be of special significance to the actor (staff nurse). The volume contains chapters on the following separate research studies: (1) A study in the nature and uses of nursing notes, (2) The accuracy of the TPR procedure, (3) Functions of the Shift Report, (4) Authority Structure, Ambiguity of the Medical Task, Absence of the Doctor from the Ward and the Behavior of Nurses, (4) An experiment in ward management, and (6) The use of discretion by nurses—doctors' expectations and nurses' perceptions. (JC)

262   PC, NR

Warstler, M. E. Some management techniques for nursing service administrators. *Journal of Nursing Administration.* Nov.-Dec. 1972, 2(6): 25–34. (See also #263)

Suggestions on how to document data for decision making and to justify needs for personnel and materials. Factors causing fluctuations in patient care are briefly described. A patient classification system for medical and surgical patients, adults and children, maternity patients, newborn infants, and psychiatric patients is outlined. Various other reports are demonstrated. Daily nursing hours for each category of patient, average and range, are described and effect of unit management briefly mentioned, as well as other factors affecting nursing hours. Not considered, due to lack of documented data, is the proportion of the determined hours needed for each classification that must be contributed by professional, technical, and auxiliary nursing personnel to achieve the desired level of quality care. (JB)

263   NR

Warstler, M. E. (ed.) *Staffing: A journal of nursing administration reader.* Wakefield, Mass.: Contemporary Publishing, Inc., 1974.

A compilation of ten previously published articles (including #015, #098, and #262) which provide a combination of "how to" articles with conceptual discussions of value to administrators. Articles are well written and provide resources to assist the reader in evaluating and analyzing needs, and implementation of staffing programs. The underlying rationales of the approaches are presented. (JB)

264   NR

Warstler, M. E. (ed.) *Staffing: A journal of nursing administration reader.* Wakefield, Mass.: Contemporary Publishing, Inc., 1974.

Process of development of the nursing practice statement adopted by the California Nurses Association at its convention in March, 1971. The statement defines two levels of nursing practice, implemental and supplemental, based on the experience and input from over 600 nurses in varied practice settings. A committee of 21 nurses developed the statement. It was adopted as a first step in a plan to implement the ANA's position paper on educational preparation for nurse practitioners and assistants to nurses, in California. (JB)

265   NAP:PN, TM

Werner, J. NAQ forum: Primary nursing: Why not? *Nursing Administration Quarterly*. Winter 1977, 1(2):85–87.

This article discusses cost effectiveness and quality issues as they related to the transition from team or functional nursing to primary nursing. She reports the following findings: (1) Primary nursing costs patients no more than other conventional nursing patterns. (2) Questionnaires given to patients upon discharge indicate that primary nursing patients responded with exceptional commendations about their nursing care. (3) Complaints about nursing staff by physicians have decreased since the implementation of primary nursing. (4) Physicians rated the quality of patient care higher since the implementation of primary nursing. No data are presented on nurse turnover. (JC)

266   NAP⁺:PN

Werner, J., et al. The Evanston story: Primary nursing comes alive. *Nursing Administration Quarterly*. Winter 1977, 1(2):9–50.

This is a series of articles written by several individuals about the implementation of module, and, then, primary nursing. Project began when a consulting firm was brought in to evaluate the functioning of various hospital departments, including nursing, and to make recommendations for change, in efforts to reduce the budget. Nursing administrators were interested in formulating a staffing and scheduling system based on patient needs. Preliminary evaluation of personnel management under the team method indicated that team nursing was neither efficient nor effective as an organizational approach. It was found that nursing assistants were giving the bulk of nursing care even though 40–60 percent of their time on duty was spent in nonproductive activity such as reading magazines and coffee breaks. The RN team leaders were working very hard but 75 percent of their time was taken up with duties away from the patient. Based on this evaluation, nursing service administrators first implemented "modular" nursing and then progressed to primary nursing. (JC)

267   NR, OS, PC, NAP⁺:CS

Whitson, B. J., Hartley, L. M. & Wolford, H. G. Complemental nursing. *American Journal of Nursing*. June 1977, 77(6):984–988.

A form of independent practice is described as conceived by its originator, experienced by a patient, and practiced by a nurse. It begins with a nurse-patient contract that assures the patient care by the same nurse throughout his prehospital, hospital, and posthospital phases. (JB)

268   NAP*:PN

Williams, L. B. Evaluation of nursing care: A primary nursing project—part 1, report of the controlled study. *Supervisor Nurse*. January 1975, 6(1):32–39. (See also #090)

Spinoff report of 1973 study in which Geraldine Felton was principal nurse researcher, "Increasing the Quality of Nursing Care by Introducing the Concept of Primary Nursing: A Model Project." Describes philosophy of nursing service, rationale for measurement instruments used in the study, and outcomes. Also discusses limitations of evaluation research. (CAL)

269   NAP:TM

Williams, M. A. The myths and assumptions about team nursing. *Nursing Forum*. 1964, 3(4):61–73.

The success of team nursing does not rest upon methods, but upon the provision to staff members of recognition, security, and a chance to experience a sense of accomplishment. Only when these basic needs are met will the staff members be free to help meet patients' needs. Team nursing has become a wordfact in too many places because the interest has been in the method and not in the examination of the assumptions upon which it is based—an examination which shows that the staff members, and especially the RNs, are often being expected to perform functions for which they have not been prepared and with which they have not been helped while on the job. (CAL)

270   PC, OS*

Wood, M. Clinical sensory deprivation: A comparative study of patients in single care and two-bed rooms. *Journal of Nursing Administration.* December 1977, 7(10):28–32.

Single care units may create unanticipated difficulties for patients and nurses. This study uses the concept of sensory deprivation to examine differences in patients' responses to single care and two-bed rooms in a community hospital. The results showed that patients in single care rooms experienced significantly more sensory disturbances than did those in two-bed rooms. (Author's abstract)

271   NR

Yamamura, D. S. *Functions and role conceptions of nursing service personnel.* Honolulu: The Territorial Commission on Nursing Education and Nursing Service, University of Hawaii, 1955.

The objectives of this project were to develop in a preliminary fashion an understanding of the social position, functions, and relationships of the nursing personel in Hawaiian hospitals; and to identify that system, the attitudes of the various classes of nursing personnel toward the functions they perform, and the social and organizational factors related to the job they perform. Those interrelated questions to which the research sought preliminary answers are enumerated as follows: (1) What are the functions performed by the various classes of personnel in the nursing service? (2) What are the attitudes of various classes of personnel toward the performance of these functions? (3) What social and organizational factors in the social system of the hospital are related to job satisfaction? (JC)

272   NR, NAP[+]:PN

Zander, K. S. Primary nursing won't work. . . unless the head nurse lets it. *Journal of Nursing Administration.* October 1977, 7(8):19–23.

Primary nursing cannot succeed on any unit whose head nurse is not committed to this system of nursing care. To lead her or his staff into primary nursing, the head nurse must accept a change in her or his own role, leadership style, and functions as unit manager. If the head nurse looks upon the transition as a challenge, as a means to personel and professional growth, she or he can make primary nursing a success. (Author's abstract)

Appendix 2
NURSING ASSIGNMENT PATTERN STUDY DESCRIPTION

The following overview describes the Nursing Assignment Pattern (NAP) study undertaken by the Nursing Department.

Study Purpose

The goal of this study is to assist the Department of Nursing in choosing the appropriate nursing assignment pattern on selected patient units, by providing tools to analyze the unit's own situation and needs. The key parts of the process are gathering relevant information and analyzing it so as to reach a decision concerning the assignment pattern appropriate to the unit.

Presently, clear definitions of nursing assignment patterns do not exist. One reason for this is the quite divergent definitions of primary nursing, case assignment nursing, team nursing, functional nursing, total patient care nursing, etc. We need a method to describe assignment patterns which is not open to interpretation. Second, we need a description that allows us to compare assignment in terms of how nurses are actually used, so that we can avoid arguments which turn on the meaning of words, rather than on genuine assignment differences. In the original work leading to this approach, University of Michigan researchers would find nurses who wanted primary nursing because they deeply believed that the planning and providing of care to a single patient should be located in a single nurse. Other nurses wanted primary nursing because they deeply believed that the responsibility for the care of a patient should be located in a single person, because

then tasks could be effectively delegated to those actually providing care and care could be monitored and evaluated. These are two very different conceptions of primary nursing. In some respects, they are more different from each other than the second is from some definitions of team nursing.

Drawing on the work of Barbara Horn and other scholars in the field of organization theory, a set of ten elements has been developed that adequately characterizes any nursing assignment pattern. These elements are those shown in Figure I:1 of this book. A nursing unit, by collecting specified data, can determine the type of assignment pattern that is *actually in use*.

It is also possible to look at *patient characteristics* and consider which elements of the nursing assignment pattern are most closely related to the needs of the patients. For example, a patient with very high psychosocial support needs may benefit tremendously from a high level of nursing care integration, that is, care provided by a single person. By contrast, the patient with multiple and complex care requirements may benefit from the care of several specialists.

Beyond this, it is also possible for the unit to consider whether, given their *nursing resources,* it would be appropriate for them to move toward greater care management integration, to a different level of care management continuity, or to a different type of intershift coordination. In short, the elements of a nursing assignment pattern can be disaggregated into the elements of importance and can be related directly to the availability and competence of the nursing resource.

A third advantage of this approach to defining nursing assignment patterns lies in the opportunity to look for the weak points, so to speak, in *organizational support*. For example, it is difficult in the extreme to have high levels of care management continuity when nurse staffing or scheduling systems provide a churning of the nursing staff within a hospital. Scheduling and staffing policy are intricately related to nursing assignment pattern decisions. If these issues are to be effectively addressed, it is necessary to have a framework within which the explicit relations may be identified, and the tradeoffs openly considered.

Study Methods

Data is gathered in the hospital and analyzed with the use of connective propositions generated from the literature.

The data collection instrument has four parts. The first part is a set of questions intended to characterize the unit's present nursing assignment pattern (NAP). The second part is intended to identify the characteristics of patients who are cared for on the unit. The third part describes the nursing resources which are accessible to the unit, and the fourth part describes the organizational support that is available to the unit from the hospital.

The literature review has resulted in an annotated bibliography of about 270 items, selected because of their potential contribution to an understanding of the linkage between patient characteristics, nursing resources, and organizational support on the one hand, and appropriate nursing assignment patterns on the other. This literature review has provided a basis for the connective propositions which translate the data into appropriate recommendations for a unit's nursing assignment pattern.

The propositions have been framed so as to link NAP variables with the three sets of basic factors which should influence them: characteristics of the patient population, nature of available nursing resources, and the organizational support available to nursing units and to the patient care process. Figure A:1 pictures this conceptual framework underlying the study. The relationship between NAP and the basic influencing factors is indicated, as is the subsequent effect of NAP on nursing standards and on outcomes.

Study Results

The study requires considerable data collection and analysis, and it will be some time before recommendations will be available for discussion and review. The study should give an excellent basis for strengthening nursing organization at the patient care level.

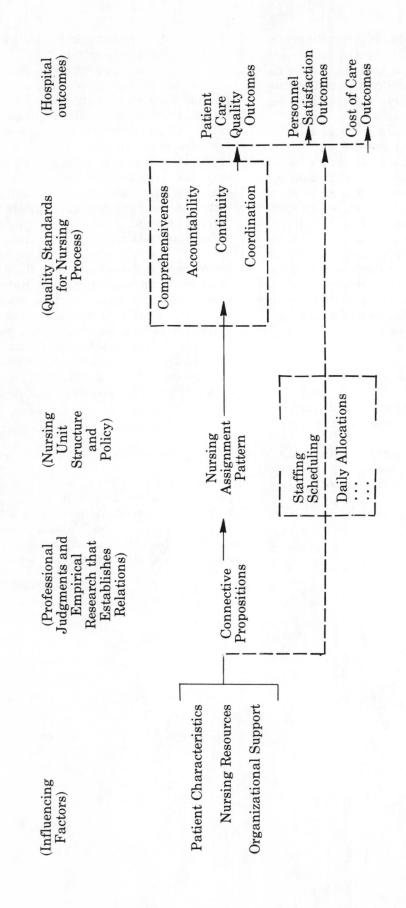

Figure A:1
Nursing Assignment Pattern
Conceptual Framework

(Influencing Factors)

Patient Characteristics
Nursing Resources
Organizational Support

Connective Propositions

(Professional Judgments and Empirical Research that Establishes Relations)

Nursing Assignment Pattern

Staffing Scheduling

Daily Allocations
. . .
. . .

(Nursing Unit Structure and Policy)

Comprehensiveness

Accountability

Continuity

Coordination

(Quality Standards for Nursing Process)

Patient Care Quality Outcomes

Personnel Satisfaction Outcomes

Cost of Care Outcomes

(Hospital outcomes)

Appendix 3

DEFINITIONS

The following definitions and assumptions were used in this manual; for definitions of variables see Figures I:1–I:4.

connective propositions—statements of the relationships between variables suggested by empirical research or professional judgments, e.g., published case studies, research studies, or reports.

nursing—a science and art whose goals are to maintain the wholeness of clients and to assist them in realizing their maximum potential, which includes health and harmonious interaction with their environment. Nursing fulfills this goal through a problem-solving process and the use of protection, nurturance, stimulation, and restoration activities in an interaction framework. (Adapted from Riehl, J. & Roy, C. *Conceptual Models for Nursing Practice* ,p. 298. New York: Appleton-Century-Crofts, 1974.)

nursing assignment pattern—the policy and structure for the assignment of nursing personnel to patient-clients for the provision of nursing care on a nursing unit.

nursing care—the application of the science and art of nursing.

nursing practice—the nursing care given by nurses and their assistants.

nursing process—the problem-solving process of assessment, planning, intervention, and evaluation applied in nursing; all of the nursing activities involved in providing care to patient-clients.

outcomes—the results or effects of the patient care structure and processes; quality of patient care, personnel satisfaction, and costs are viewed as the major outcomes related to nursing assignment patterns.

process requirements—common conditions or needs of clients requiring nursing knowledge and skills to assess, plan, intervene, and evaluate; i.e., common nursing "problems" or "diagnoses."

therapy requirements—common therapies performed by or in collaboration with nursing personnel.

Appendix 4

INDEX TO ELEMENTS AND VARIABLES

Appendix 5

REQUEST FOR USER FEEDBACK

To users of this manual, we want your help!

We expect to continue our work in developing tools for nursing managers. You can help us in three important ways:

1. By sending us comments and suggestions for improving this manual, noting errors and the ease or difficulty of using the manual (especially the instruments, coding instructions, and connective propositions). Of course, we would also appreciate positive feedback, so we know what was helpful and what we won't need to change.

2. By sharing your data with us, particularly any of the four Display Sheets that summarize your analysis, and letting us know what assignment pattern changes you made.

3. By letting us know what other uses you made of the instruments (e.g., using the satisfaction instrument in a morale survey, the patient characteristics instrument as part of a staffing analysis, etc.).

Send comments, with your name, hospital, and address, to:

Professor Fred Munson   OR   Professor Lillian Simms
School of Public Health   School of Nursing
University of Michigan   University of Michigan
Ann Arbor, Michigan 48109   Ann Arbor, Michigan 48109

THANK YOU for your time and effort!

About the Authors

Fred C. Munson, Ph.D., is Professor of Hospital Administration and Research Associate in Population Planning at the School of Public Health, University of Michigan. Professor Munson is the author of numerous articles, was co-editor of *Cost Control in Hospitals*, and has contributed chapters to several other health-related publications.

Joanne Shultz Beckman, B.S.N., M.S., is Director of the Quality Assurance Program in Nursing at Duke University Hospitals. Ms. Beckman was formerly a lecturer and clinical supervisor at the University of Michigan, School of Nursing, and contributed to a two-volume HEW manual entitled *Development of Criterion Measures of Nursing Care*.

Jacqueline Clinton, M.A., R.N., is a Ph.D. candidate at the University of Michigan, School of Nursing, and has served as Nursing Consultant/Data Analyst for the Michigan Department of Mental Health. Ms. Clinton was an Assistant Professor of Nursing at Bowling Green State University and a Clinical Nursing Specialist for the Veterans Administration in Wichita, Kansas.

Carolyn Kever, S.S.N., M.P.H., is an Assistant Administrator at the Kaiser-Permanente Medical Center in Santa Clara, California. Her professional experience combines extensive research with clinical and supervisory nursing skills.

Lillian M. Simms., R.N., Ph.D., is an Associate Professor of Nursing and Director for the Graduate Program in Nursing Health Services Administration, School of Nursing, University of Michigan, and recent (1978) co-author of *The Nurse Person: Perspectives for Contemporary Nursing*.